Benedict Nta Tanka's Commentary and dramatized ideas on
"Disease and Witchcraft in our Society"

Medizin in Entwicklungsländern

Schriftenreihe zur Medizin und zu Gesundheitsproblemen in Ländern der Dritten Welt

Herausgegeben von
Prof. Dr. med. Hans Jochen Diesfeld, Heidelberg

In Fortführung der Schriftenreihe „Gesundheitsprobleme in Entwicklungsländern“
der Lehranstalt für Allgemein- und Sozialhygiene an der Universität Hamburg
Herausgegeben von Prof. (em.) Dr. med. Habil. Dr. phil. H. Harmsen

Band 7

Verlag Peter D. Lang
Frankfurt a.M. • Bern • Cirencester/U.K.

Alexander Boroffka

Benedict Nta Tanka's Commentary and Dramatized Ideas on »Disease and Witchcraft in our Society«

A Schreber Case from Cameroon
Annotated Autobiographical Notes
by an African on his Mental Illness

Verlag Peter D. Lang
Frankfurt a.M. • Bern • Cirencester/U.K.

CIP-Kurztitelaufnahme der Deutschen Bibliothek

*** Nta Tanka, Benedict:**

[Commentary and dramatized ideas on "Disease and witchcraft in our society"]
Benedict Nta Tanka's commentary and dramatized ideas on "Disease and witchcraft in our society" : a Schreber case from Cameroon annotated auto= biograph. notes by an African on his mental illness / Alexander Boroffka. - Frankfurt a.M., Bern, Cirencester/U.K. : Lang, 1980.
(Medizin in Entwicklungsländern ; Bd. 7)
ISBN 3-8204-6901-X
NE: Boroffka, Alexander [Hrsg.]

ISBN 3-8204-6901-X

Druck: fotokop Wilhelm Weihert KG, Darmstadt

To Nora

PREFACE

by

Professor T. Adeoye Lambo, M.D., F.R.C.P., F.R.C.Psy., Hon.DSc., Hon.LLD.; Deputy Director-General, World Health Organization
Formerly Professor of Psychiatry, University of Ibadan, Nigeria

Kierkegaard had said that the study of aberration should lead to a better understanding of the norm. Autobiographical accounts by individuals who had experienced episodes of mental illness have certainly contributed much to our knowledge of the workings of the human mind, even if their help in unraveling the causes of mental disorders has been modest. The modern obsession with sample sizes, controlled trials and tests of statistical significance, all necessary scientific tools of medicine - has tended to obscure to a certain extent the less glamorous but uniquely rewarding pathway to knowledge in psychiatry, the painstaking in-depth study of the individual case.

The annotated autobiographical notes of Mr. Benedict Nta Tanka, a 37-year old civil servant in Cameroon, presented and commented upon in this volume by Alexander Boroffka, make a document of considerable significance. They illustrate in great and vivid detail the inner dialectics of a personality confronting a mental illness which, by all the clinical evidence, could be diagnosed as a paranoid form of schizophrenia. The account, however, is much more than a mere illustration of the applicability of customary diagnostic criteria in the context of an African culture.

Mr. Tanka's experiences bring across to the reader with unusual clarity the complex interplay of unintelligible, primary mental contents produced by the illness itself, and the internalized system of beliefs, attitudes and norms of his culture which has its roots in a tribal faith, moulded by the trials and passions of a singularly religious people. In African philosophies and religions, existence, and not events is the subject of their primary interest; they represent a cosmology, not a story. They put man in the centre of the universe and make the stars circle about him and this must have some kind of justification. And indeed, its justification (if I may be so brief on so great a subject) is that what is false in the science of facts may be true in the science of values.

Above all, however, the autobiographical notes witness an exceptionally strong urge to come to terms with the mental turmoil caused by the illness and to re-establish in Mr. Tanka's subjective perception the objective harmony of the world in which the traditional African society believes. In a very large measure Benedict Tanke has succeeded in this.

In this country, i.e. Africa, the distant past has a charismatic aura and forms the basis of life and legacy of man. In recent times the decline of traditional norms, which undermined the true development of man, has become a painful reality to many. The African continent remains a cosmos which derives its strength and weakness from the richness of its profound diversity of culture, religion, politics, ethics, belief systems, and social tradition; a continent in which negative and positive influences merge in a state of anxious concern.

Undoubtedly, the pharmacological treatment has helped Mr. Tanka's recovery. To what an extent, however, his personality make-up and the cosmology that pervades his view of himself, the others and the world, have played a role in his recovery? This is difficult to answer scientifically in the individual case but is a fascinating subject for further research. If the important finding of the WHO International Pilot Study of Schizophrenia that schizophrenic psychoses in Africans tended to have better outcome than clinically comparable schizophrenic disorders in Europeans and North Americans is further confirmed, the study of the factors responsible for such differences may become one of the most promising leads to the understanding of the nature of this prevalent and frequently devastating disease. Individual case studies like the one presented in this volume should complement the epidemiological, clinical and biological approaches.

Alexander Boroffka was Professor of Psychiatry at the University of Ibadan, Nigeria, and has had extensive experience in Africa. He is pre-eminent in his diagnosis and total therapeutic management of the African patient; his regard for the culture and his sensitivity to psychodynamic interpretation of events within the African context is almost unrivalled. This work will stand as a historical monument in the history of psychiatry, being the first to be described in non-literate cultures after the celebrated Freud's Schreber case.

There is, lastly, another aspect to Mr. Tanka's testimony presented in this book. Being the first extensive autobiographical document of this kind written by a non-European, it is a reminder of the basic unity of Man across cultures and epochs. Clinical details apart, the existential reasons for Mr. Tanka's dramatization of a segment of his life are not very dissimilar to those of Kierkegaard's: transcedence of personal suffering through search for universals.

Mr. Tanka's experience has once again shown that in the distant past, in the phenomenon of ancestor-worship and supernaturalism was the transcript of the real experience of humanity, as men found it in their innermost souls and as they were dimly aware of it in universal history. It carried the imagination into a new phase; it sanctified the poverty and sorrow at which Western religion had shuddered; it awakened tender emotions, revealed more human objects of adoration and furnished subtle instruments of grace. This spiritual world constituted a system complete and consistent within itself. There was occasion within it for the exercise of reason, for the awakening and discipline of emotion, for the exertion of effort. In all this, there is a lesson for the theory and practice of psychiatry.

TABLE OF CONTENTS

1. FOREWORD

Many accounts of schizophrenic illness have been written by patients. Psychiatrists, especially the ones with experience in institutions caring for the chronically ill, are often familiar with autobiographical writings of this type. Few of these writings are easy to read because of the way in which they are presented. Often it is extremely difficult and time consuming to understand, or, even vaguely, to follow the meanderings of the disturbed mind. Very often also the quality of the style makes it unattractive to delve into it.

No wonder then, that few of these documents have been published. Some have been printed since their authors could afford to pay for it but mostly they have soon disappeared again in oblivity (Spiess, 1966). Maybe the most famous publication of this kind is Schreber's "Memoirs of my Nervous Illness" (Schreber, 1973; Macalpine and Hunter, 1955), famous mainly because Sigmund Freud used it as material for his hypotheses on paranoia, published in 1911. These hypotheses have been discussed ever since. They have made the autobiography world famous as its translation into English convincingly proves. But it is not only of interest to the psychiatric historian. In addition to this side, the book gives innumerable examples of the ways how the schizophrenic mind works which no textbook can equate.

Finally the writing has some quality of style which sometimes also can be found in productions of schizophrenics. It exerts a strong aesthetic attraction and, whilst reading the book, instruction is combined with a certain intellectual pleasure and stimulation. That this quality of "schizophrenic thinking" can be found in patients the world around is accepted by most scholars nowadays. I do not know of any more striking characterization of the schizophrenic ways of behaviour, not only of the schizophrenic thinking, as those given by Vyncke (1958) describing African patients suffering from this condition:

> "Nous avons entendu de la bouche de nos schizophrènes africains parfois textuellement les mêmes phrases que chez les schizophrènes d'Europe, parfois même nous avons trouvé les mêmes dessins, et parfois aussi ce même sourire guindé de la "Joconde" de da Vinci, sans parler de tant d'autres attitudes et comportements typiquement schizophrènes et qui se révélaient tous être étrangement les mêmes ici et en Europe. "

The direct obersvation of the similarity of the schizophrenic thinking in patients from different creeds and cultures has been limited to psychiatrists who had a chance to work in different countries or continents. The author was not able to locate a single publication of an extensive case study of an African suffering from schizophrenic disorder which would make this observation possible for scientists not being able to treat patients from outside the Western world.

The fashion of the day are epidemiological studies in which relatively few single facts on a very large number of patients are collected and analysed. The previous extreme, the fashion of our psychiatric grandfathers, like Kraepelin or Adolph Mayer, to collect life histories of single patients and using a descriptive analysis, has been neglected in modern psychiatric writing. Not many psychiatrists in training and afterwards, when travelling up and down the countries to fulfil their functions as social and home visiting psychiatrists, or when concerned with drugs, studying the latest releases of our all too eager drug companies, will find the time and leisure to prepare and analyse extensive case studies of single patients.

It was a stroke of luck that Mr. Benedict Tanka in the first instance wrote down his experiences during a severe psychotic episode; that secondly, he had very understanding supervisors and doctors who referred him finally for psychiatric treatment and made the desirable follow-up possible; and thirdly, that the attending psychiatrist was not only interested in the patient's writings but, due to unforseeable personal circumstances, found himself in a position to spare the time necessary to prepare the writings for publication.

Thus, this "African Schreber Case" is presented to the reader.

The volume makes available for the first time a full account of a paranoid schizophrenic psychosis in an African patient who, could one have wished for more co-indidence?, is also the first literate member in his whole family. In so far it is already a curiosum as such. But in addition, the case study demonstrates, after a very serious beginning, at least very serious according to Western standards, the rather benign course of the illness for the nine years during which the editor was able to follow up the patient. This unusual course of the illness might be a characteristic of the African, as many more similar cases of the same benign course in undoubtable schizophrenics have been observed (WHO, 1973; 1979).

The last but not the least feature of these documents is their literary quality which, in the opinion of the editor, provides a unique reading experience. It makes possible insight into an exotic world populated by spirits, influenced by the super-imposition of some facets of the Western world which have or are about to disappear already in the West, which are seen through the searching eyes of a young man, although handicapped temporarily by mental disorder but nervertheless keen to grasp the meaning of the world in which he lives and which seems to pose the question to him:

Illness or Preconceived?

2. INTRODUCTION

THE SEQUENCE OF PRESENTATION

The main content of this volume are the writings of Mr. Benedict Tanka, a Cameroonian, born 1943, who was twenty-five years old when he became ill. Two and a half years later he was referred to the Department of Psychiatry, University College Hospital, Ibadan, Nigeria, where he presented some of his writings; others were sent by letters from 1974 to 1979.

Preceding Mr. T.'s writings, in 3. Clinical Notes, a full case history is given as it was collected during his stay at the hospital from 25th September, 1970 to 22nd December, 1970 and at his two follow-up visits in 1971 and 1972. The case study includes history, findings, therapy, course of illness, and previous medical reports.

The order of 4. Writings of Mr. B. N. Tanka follows the sequence in which he had written them originally.

In Part I, Mr. T. gives an exact description of his psychotic experiences which began on 19th March, 1968. He tries to explain these events as consequences of witchcraft. The introduction discusses the possibilities of illness and witchcraft both causing suffering to man. The end of Part I takes up again more general ideas whereas the main part is concerned with the subtle description of all the hallucinatory and delusional experiences. Mr. T. wrote Part I during the month of February 1969. He wrote it in long-hand and had it later typed by a typist.

In Part II, the events described in Part I are partly repeated; some are supplemented and some are elaborated. The fasicinating side of this part is the transformation of the whole episode into something which Mr. T. calls a play. According to his explanations, the play covers the period from March 1968 until April 1970. He had started to write the play in February 1970, continued during March and completed it in April 1970. He wrote it, like Part I, in longhand and had it later typed by a typist. When comparing Part I and Part II it seems, that Mr. T., when writing the play about a year later, had already gained some distance to the originally very frightening experiences. The play has a distinct meaning for him and he calls it a tragedy in the beginning which turns later on into a comedy in the end (see footnote 59).

Part III was written during the first weeks of September 1970 just preceding his attendance to the hospital in preparation of his journey to Ibadan. It is the summary of Part I and II in the form of eighty relatively short paragraphs which, so he explained, he prepared to make the reading easier and less time consuming for the doctors. He was afraid they would not be able and willing to read carefully through the eighty-three foolscap pages of his original manuscripts which contained somewhat over forty thousand words. Part III gives the reader a good opportunity to become familiar with the style, the personality and the experiences of Mr. Tanka. Since no new facts are described and no new formulations are being used no further annotations have been added. It might be useful to read this summary before the main parts.

Part IV contains 58 dreams. Thirty-eight were collected and written down by Mr. Tanka on request of a previous doctor in 1968, who had the hand-written notes typed. Mr. Tanka handed a copy of this script to me in 1970 together with his other writings. It was not possible to talk with Mr. T. about the dreams and to record free associations in connection with the dreams, due to lack of time, but also because Mr.T. was somewhat reluctant to discuss the dreams, different from his willingness to discuss his other writings. The additional twenty dreams, some of them dated, were sent together with a letter in 1979.

Part V consists of the excerpted and partly edited writings I have received from Mr. Tanka since March 1974 until 1979, containing numerous letters, filled in questionnaires in regard of the development of his condition and descriptions in regard of his tribe.

THE EDITING

Generally the orthography of the patient was kept and as little alterations as possible were made. Some minor alterations were necessary in order to make the text understandable for the reader. These alterations consisted of changing capital letters into small ones and vice versa, in the adjustment of some of the punctuation, and finally in correcting some obvious spelling mistakes. In the latter the editor was trying to follow the line of corrections the patient himself had applied when he corrected the copy which was typed by somebody else and from which our copy was retyped. In a number of cases it remained dubious if a certain spelling is intention and might indicate thought disorder or neologism, or if it is just weakness in orthography; examples of both are indicated in the annotations.

THE ANNOTATIONS

When Part I and Part II were handed over to the editor by the patient, which happened only after he had been on the ward already for some weeks, the editor read them marking obscure expressions or words and sentences, requiring explanation. These passages were then discussed with Mr. T. His comments were taken down and constitute most of the footnotes. They are always put in quotation marks when presented literally. Some of the notes refer to certain psychopathological phenomena and, although rarely, to possible interpretations or hidden meanings.

Although the patient stayed in Ibadan for almost three months - the time which the editor was able to spend with him was necessarily limited due to the editor's duties in the department which were especially heavy during those months. Many passages remain, in which further clarification by the patient would have been desirable. From the beginning, the editor was aware of this situation. He was confronted with two alternatives. Either he had to give up the whole idea of making these unique documents available to the profession, or he had to publish them in their necessarily incomplete form. The latter alternative was chosen since it was possible to present the writings of Mr. T. in full, even if some explanations may be lacking. To accomplish even this task was not easy for a sparsely staffed overworked office as every page had to be retyped during a few weeks as the patient, understandably, wanted to take his copies with him on his departure.

MR. B. TANKA'S OPINION IN REGARD OF PUBLICATION

When I first discussed with Mr. T. the possibility that his writings might be of interest to a wider readership he was very keen on this idea. He fully agreed with a publication which he confirmed in signing a statement to this extent. He further insisted that neither his name, nor any other name, nor any of the circumstances or dates should be changed. Mr. Tanka may be quoted himself from paragraph 1, Part I: "In writing this story I have made mention of some names. Some of which are names of persons still living or dead and the rest are names which I knew when the incidents occured. As this is a story that may be teaching to each and everyone of us, I plead to those whose names appear in this story from time to time, not to be upset."

The editor wants to join this appeal whole heartedly. Although at first he was somewhat hesitant about Mr. T's insistence in this respect, he finally felt compelled and even obliged to follow Mr. T's instructions to the word, not changing anything. The editor is confident that it will be obvious to every person be he or she well known in public or not, that their names, and the actions ascribed to them are only and merely occurring within the thinking of Mr. T. Anybody familiar with psychiatry will recognize immediately by reading these chapters - and any other interested reader may be honestly assured of it - that these events are not describing events having occured in reality to the personalities mentioned; their reality lies in Mr. T's thinking, experiences and perceptions.

3. CLINICAL NOTES

REASON FOR ADMISSION

Mr. Benedict N. Tanka, a Cameroonian, 27 years old, reported at the Psychiatric Clinic of the University College Hospital, Ibadan, on 25 September, 1970. There had been no advance notification of his arrival nor did he bring any referral note from his previous doctors or his Government in the Cameroons from wehre he had arrived the previous day. He had with him several medical reports from 1968 and 1969 according to which he had suffered from a mental disorder since March 1968. The medical reports are reproduced at the end of this chapter.

The patient was seen by the consultant and by the psychiatric social worker. The patient reported that he was experiencing voices commenting on his thoughts and at times telling him what to do. He feels a group of people in his home country are responsible for these experiences. He referred to his writing in regard of these occurences. He also complained of crawling or piercing sensations all over his body, sleepiness and general weakness of the body.

The patient did not know anybody in Ibadan or environs. He did not have sufficient means to maintain himself. He assured the hospital authorities that his government would be responsible for the hospital bill, which proved later on to be correct. Consequently it was not possible to consider out-patient treatment. Mr. T. himself felt in need of help and wanted to be admitted although he was convinced of the reality of his experiences which he did not consider as signs of illness. Since the need for intensive psychiatric treatment was obvious, the patient was admitted, as soon as a bed became vacant, on 28 September, 1970, to a general medical ward where the beds of the Department for male psychiatric patiens were available.

All information on the patient comes from himself and from the short medical certificates mentioned previously.

(a) CASE HISTORY

Family History:

Benedict Tanka comes from a poor family of small farmers. He belongs to the Menka, a small tribe living in the coastal belt of rain forests in the Western Cameroons (see Part V). He does not know much about his ancestors. None of his grandparents are alive. He remembers one grandmother who also appears in his writings. His forefathers, as far as he knows, have all been farmers living in and around his home village. Both parents are alive and healthy. Both had no chance to attend any school. They are both Christians but were converted to Christianity only as adults.

The father is about 50 years old (but see following paragraph). Besides subsistence farming, he is producing some palm oil from which he draws a small income. Thereby it was possible for him to help the patient through his school education.

The patient's mother is his father's senior wife. According to the patient she is somewhat over forty years old. Early marriage for girls is the rule, but she must have been at least sixteen or seventeen years old when she delivered her first child. This puts her age at about 48 years now. Consequently it must be assumed that the patient's father is rather close to sixty years and not fifty as stated. A junior wife, and the widow of a deceased brother of the father are living with the father as his second and third wives, which is the custom of many ethnical groups in West Africa.

All three wives have children of their own, but only two have borne their children to Mr. T.'s father. Patient's mother has borne six children:

1. Male child, born around 1938, died as a baby.
2. Male child, born 1939, had very little schooling, is working as farmer; he is married with children.
3. Patient, born 1943.
4. Female, born 1946, married, has three children; no schooling.
5. Female, born 1949, married,has one child; no schooling.
6. Female, born 1952, married, has one child; educated up to Primary School, Class VI.

The patient is certain that there was, and is no mental illness in his family, neither on his father's nor his mother's side. Patient feels he has always been on good terms with all members of his family. There has also been and still is a good relationship between his parents. The polygamous way of life taken over from the ancestors does not prevent his parents from being devoted Christians. They belong to the Roman Catholic church. At first the patient had reported to the European editor that his parents lived in a monogamous marriage. The polygamous family structure was reported as a matter of fact to the Nigerian social worker but was not kept a secret any longer in later interviews with the editor.

Personal History:

Mr. T. was born in 1943. He does not know date or month of his birth. He knows from his mother that he was a very sickly child. He suffered from yaws which left scars on his arms. He needed a lot of looking after. In later years he has never been ill and did not need any medical treatment. He was baptised a Roman Catholic Christian in 1949 when he started his primary education. Except for a short period of schooling of his surviving elder brother, the patient was the very first person of his family who had received a formal education. Later his youngest sister completed Primary school but did not go any further. After his primary school, Mr. T. attended a Secondary School from 1955 to 1961. He completed Class 5 but failed to obtain the West African School Certificate. This was a heavy blow to him, and to his family as well, since a lot was and still is expected from him. He tried once again to take the '0' level Examination of the General Certificate of Education but was not successful.

In March 1962 he started work as a Clerk in the Department of Education. He still is in the same Department. At the beginning of his illness he was living and working at Kumba; at present he is posted to the Education Office in Buea, Western Cameroons. He passed his promotion examination in July 1966 and was promoted Second Class Clerk, which post he is still holding. Many of his old schoolmates and colleagues have superseded him at work. Many have graduated and are in well paid jobs. The patient does not worry much about this and moves freely with his old friends.

Before his illness started he was about to marry a girl named Rose, who figures prominently in his writings. The patient feels that the girl did not behave in the same way, after his illness started, as she did before. So he does not really know what is going to happen with his relationship. The girl Rose had gone to Britain for further education in 1964 after they had known each other for a long time. She came back only in September 1968, teaching in school as a domestic science mistress. Since then he had noticed her change of behaviour.

Patient was very shy and reluctant to talk about sexual inclinations and practices. He did convey, but without stating it explicitly, that he has had no actual sexual experience because it was considered as wrong by his church. From information obtained from other African patients, less prudish than Mr. T., one could infer that a short lasting period of masturbation, followed by occasional play with girls is quite usual during adolescence but not necessarily for the adult young man. For Mr. T. the moral climate in his family is decisive and there is no reason not to believe the impressions conveyed by the patient. In his writings though, there are several references to sexual matters and on two occasions he stated that he had dreams about sexual contents and that he regards such dreams as dreadful "because he could not sleep".

Before March 1968 patient reports that he had never had any nervous or mental trouble or any other serious disease.

Actually no more information on the patient's previous personality could be extracted from him. He sees himself as a sociable, moderately ambitious and generally happy person. He had few hobbies but spent quite some time with his friends. He considered himself as a rather calm and stable but generally cheerful person. All this has changed since his present illness began.

Present Illness:

His illness started exactly at 8 p.m. on 19 March 1968. Patient's very extensive written descriptions are available to the reader in the following chapters. Most of his narratives during several interviews followed closely, even literally, these written accounts. His illness started with voices giving him orders, commenting on his thoughts and putting thoughts into his mind.

He was first seen and treated by the Area Medical Officer in Tiko Hospital near Kumba, Dr. Lantum, who diagnosed a paranoid schizophrenia, prescribed a sedative and vitamins, and on 18 April 1968, referred him to a Mission Hospital near Bamenda for further treatment since he was to spend his leave near that place at his home village.

Dr. Schwarz from Acha Tugi Hospital in his report of 7 May, 1968, confirms the original diagnosis: he found the "Rorschach Psychodiagnostic Test not very pathological." He prescribed permanent sleep therapy with daily injections of a psycholepticum for a week, had personal interviews with the patient, and referred to the patient's dreams (included in this volume as Part IV). The patient complained of sleeplessness and was advised to postpone his studies for the General Certificate of Education. Continuation of neuroleptic drugs and a hypnotic was suggested.

On 17 June 1968, Dr. Lantum discharged the patient from sick leave but recommended light duties and a transfer since his previous environment might "precipitate his old condition". However, the transfer did not take place for some time and Mr. T. continued his work in Kumba.

There is another medical report by Dr. Schwarz, dated 6 December 1968 in which Mr. T. is considered "bodily fit to undergo the training course without physical exercices, farm work and sports. Mental difficulties are likely to occur".

In early 1969, according to the patient, he was transfered to Bamenda. But this transfer did not improve his condition. The previous experiences returned and even became stronger. It seems that he had to go on sick leave again in August 1969 as the Medical Officer in charge of the General Hospital in Bamenda reported on 4 November 1969 that he has "been following Mr. T. medically since August 22, 1969, that he is much better and that he can return to light duties."

Although his psychotic experiences continued, Mr. T. seems to have managed to stay at his post. In early 1970 he was transferred again, this time to Buea. He continued some treatment although there are no further medical reports available after December 1969, although from the reports it seems that he must have suffered from severe psychotic symptoms most of the time. He finally convinced his supervisors to send him for intensive psychiatric treatment to Ibadan, Nigeria, more than 600 km away. It was later explained by a letter from his Ministry that the patient had not waited for the referral letter by his attending doctor; once the permission was given he set out on his own and came to Ibadan on 25 September 1970 without the proper documents to support his request for treatment. Considering his personality this is but another proof how much he must have suffered.

When comparing Mr. T.'s written report and his statements at the various interviews it seems, that for some months already preceding his admission, there was a change of some of the symptoms. What originally had been definite and obvious tactile hallucinations, experienced in connection with the spirits entering and leaving his body, developed gradually more into a hypochondrical quality. When Mr. T. reported at the clinic he complained of crawling, pinching sensations in his chest, and of other somatic, or rather psychosomatic, complaints, as general weakness, sleepiness and sleeplessness.

Summary of History:

Without indication of previous mental disorder or of any nervous trouble in the family, Mr. T. fell suddenly ill, at the age of 25, in March 1968. A schizophrenia, paranoid type was diagnosed. He underwent several courses of treatment by physicians and also by traditional healers; he was put on extended periods of sick leave at least twice, and was finally referred to the University College Hospital, Ibadan, as his symptoms and complaints did not disappear.

Physical State:

Mr. T. is a young man of slightly under average height. His weight of about 60 kilograms corresponds to his height. He is in reasonably good nutritional and general condition.

The physical examination did not reveal any abnormalities. There were a few superficial scars, some on the arms, which were explained by the patient as residuals from the yaws he had suffered in childhood; other scars on the upper back, on the chest and on both wrists and one at the back of the right foot were caused, according to the patient, by cuts administered by traditional healers.

The routine laboratory tests were within normal limits; the V. D. R. L. test was negative.

Mental Status:

The patient is fully conscious and orientated in all qualities. He is able to look after himself and to complete difficult tasks as shown by the fact, that he just had managed to travel to a foreign country, more than six-hundred kilometres from his home, changing planes, using taxis etc. He is very well able to give a full report of his experiences in the past and at present. From the beginning he seems to be very eager to get medical help but not for his psychotic experiences, which appear absolutely real to him, but rather for the detrimental consequences of these experiences on his health.

When discussing this point, the patient starts reasoning in a paralogical way. There is also indication of ambivalence. His thought process, on the surface, seems quite reasonable but if one comes near his psychotic experiences, his thinking becomes slightly unreasonable, paralogical, and unusual associations can be observed.

When asked, he describes that he is hearing voices which are giving commands or are commenting on his thoughts. Other thoughts are put into his mind. People are talking about him, behind his back and also openly. His thoughts are spoken aloud. Disconnected ideas were put together through alliteration and loose associations. Sometimes he talks beside the point and sometimes does not grasp the essential nature of an issue.

He is seeing strange visions. Some of the "spirits" in form of flies are entering his body and are causing many different distinct and very unusual feelings. At one time he smelt a very bad odour. There was never any bad or unusual taste.

All these experiences are caused by a large number of people, some known to him, some not known. It must be a kind of conspiration; although he has never found out what really is behind these occurences.

At times he feels a very important person. Religious connotations are present as well.

His mood is rather calm and even, but appears somewhat inadequate when considering it in connection with the above experiences which really must be frightening.

On the ward he keeps mostly to himself: when talked to he is very eager to discuss his condition and especially his physical complaints. He shows little or no initiative to communicate with other patients or the staff of the general medical ward.

His memory is very acute; his recall excellent for every minor fact from history and especially from his psychotic experiences.

His intelligence and general information is appropriate to his educational and cultural background and of average level.

His writings show a peculiar mixture between a very good command of rare words in English and, on the other hand, a gross misspelling of some words. Some of it can only be explained as part of his thinking disorder.

Certainly the most prominent features of this patient are his writings which depict his mental status in such a magnificent way that every attempt to describe it must appear somewhat feeble in comparison.

The patient's written account of his illness, presented in three different versions, gives examples of a multitude of different symptoms and it would require the quotation of long passages of psychiatric textbooks to accomplish an exhaustive description. This, of course, is one of the reasons for making his descriptions available in full.

The last item to be discussed under the heading of Mental Status is insight and judgement. The best way to assess these qualities is by describing them as ambivalent. The patient does not doubt in the least the reality of his visions, of the voices and of his other experiences; and still, he has been travelling from one doctor to another in order to obtain effective medical attention.

Summary of findings and diagnostic considerations:

This 27-year old male patient, the first one literate from a traditional, healthy family of farmers, who has been sickly as a child and who has suffered from yaws but otherwise had never been ill, suddenly in March 1968 developed a psychotic disorder which has been continuing with some variations of intensity until his admission in September 1970. The disorder was characterised by thought disorder of different types, including neologisms, écho de pensée, and thoughts being put into his mind. It included auditory, visual, tactile and olfactory hallucinations. There were a certain inadequateness of affect and also delusions of persecution, of grandeur, of religious and, possibly, of sexual content.

There is no indication of any physical abnormality. The very prominence of the thought disorder excludes paranoia; the length of time passed since the beginning of the illness excludes a paranoid reaction of the bouffé délirante or any other type. The most likely diagnosis was, and had already been made at the beginning of his illness by the first attending physician:

Diagnosis:

Paranoid Schizophrenia.

Therapy and course of illness:

It was clear from the beginning that, after a history of more than two years, intensive treatment would be required. In order not to disturb the communication with the patient and the development of his own insight, we refrained from ECT and, as it turned out, there was no need for it. He was first tried on thioridazine and chlorpromazine (both in high doses). But there was very little change. After two weeks treatment was changed to trifluperazine. Whilst gradually reducing the dose of chlorpromazine, trifluperazine was increased up to 10 mg t. d. s. Whilst in the hospital the patient was seen regularly by the editor, by the Registrar and by the Social Worker. Supportive psychotherapy was applied throughout the time of his stay. Since the middle of November the psychotic experiences gradually were fading away. On 12 November 1970 the patient reported that there were no more hallucinations. His delusions also became more unreal to him. Although it is difficult to put down a specific date, one could say, from around 20 November there were no more psychotic experiences. Patient's writings were discussed with him and it was amazing and interesting to note how he developed gradually an ability to point out his psychotic ways of thinking which he fully recognized as such.

Discharge was gradually being discussed with the patient and finally fixed for the week before Christmas.

Patient was discharged on 22 December 1970, after having been on the ward for almost three months. During the intensive treatment all psychotic symptoms had disappeared and the patient had gradually developed insight into the pathological nature of his experiences. Except for occasional physical complaints of different types not explained by any organic pathology, a slight remaining vagueness in his activities and a hardly noticeable flatness or rather unconcernedness of mood, the final interviews did not reveal any abnormal symptoms or signs. On discharge patient received trifluperazine 5 mg.t. d. s., chloropromazine 100 mg. nocte, benzhexol 2 mg. t. d. s. and chlordiazepoxide 10 mg. twice daily. In his final report it was recommended to reduce this drug regime to trifluperazine 5 mg. in the morning, chloropromazine 100 mg. at night and benzhexol 2 mg. twice daily.

(b) Follow-up:

After his discharge, until his next visit to the department in August 1971, the patient wrote five letters to the editor. He was not able to continue the prescribed medication since trifluperazine was not obtainable. Thus he had to continue on chloropromazine alone, after the supply of trifluperazine provided by the hospital had run out. In February 1971 the voices appeared again; in March, besides the voices, some vague physical complaints came again to the fore. However, with the drugs available, the patient managed to continue with his job. The attending physician in Victoria reported by letter of 18 June 1971 of the patient's satisfactory progress and also occasionally returning symptoms of the previous type (see annex.).

Mr. Tanka reported in Ibadan on the agreed day in August 1971. He repeated the information that the voices had been present since they had reappeared in February; but he did not pay much attention to them although he mused once again who the originators of the voices could be and for what purpose he was worried by them. During the last few weeks before his visit they had slightly diminished.

Besides an increase of chloropromazine (100 b. d.) and chlordiazepoxide 10 mg. at night, the patient was started on triperidol, the dose gradually increasing to 2 x 5 drops (= 0. 25 mg.b. d.). A sufficient supply for eleven months was given to the patient.

There were no letters from the patient until he reported again on 11 July 1972. At his visit the patient was perfectly well. There was no indication of the previous psychotic symptoms, no hallucinations, no thinking disorder. His affect was adequate to the situation. He was happy with his work and did not experience any difficulties although he had not been promoted yet. In December 1971 he had married a 18-year old girl from his home village, selected by his family. He did not know her before. He is very happy with her. She is now pregnant. He continues to attend his church services regularly. He maintains to be a happy and healthy man.

He has taken his drugs regularly. Throughout those eleven months there were none of the previous experiences.

When examined there was a slight twitching of the mouth. Since this could be a side effect of neuroleptic drugs, an increase of benzhexol was prescribed and chloropromazine was reduced to 100 mg. at night. The patient was advised to continue triperidol until the supply would be exhausted after about four weeks. After that he should start pimozide 4 mg. daily, since samples of the other drug were not available.

In February 1973, the patient wrote a letter to confirm his appointment for July 1973. According to this letter he was only suffering from occasional backache; otherwise he continued to feel perfectly well; none of the previous experiences had returned.

The patient was not able to visit Ibadan in 1973. Therefore the original follow-up ends here.

The continuation of the follow-up, from 1974 to 1980, will be found in chapter 6, taking further writings of Mr. Tanka into consideration.

Summary

Mr. Tanka suffered from a psychosis which took a rather violent course for about two years, but had quietened down somethat before he attended the University College Hospital in Ibadan. After intensive neuroleptic treatment was started, supported by social and psycho-therapy, the symptoms disappeared temporarily for the first time in more than two and a half years.

After some drugs could not be continued symptoms reappeared, until a neuroleptic drug of the butyrophenone group was introduced. From August 1971 until early 1973, the time of writing this preliminary summary, the patient had been completely free of symptoms. He was able to maintain his job and was considered cured by his family who selected a wife for him.

All this time the patient had been under a maintenance medication. The prognosis at that time was considered as rather favourable. The continuation of the follow-up, which was carried out by correspondence only, beginning March 1974 and continued until the present time (1979), will follow the writings of Mr. Tanka and forms Chapter 6.4.

(c) Annexes, Medical Reports

Dr. Dan N. Lantum, Area Medical Officer, Tiko Hospital: Letter to The Medical Officer in charge, Acha-Tugi Hospital of 18th April, 1968: "This client of ours is on leave at Gwofon and we are referring him to you for further treatment. He is a Civil Servant in the category of clerk in the Education Office, Kumba.

He has marked signs and symptoms of Schizophrenia Paranoid. He is on Oblivion Capsules, Phenobarb, Tabs. Multivite. Kindly look after him during his two months leave and communicate us of clinical developments when he is returning to the south."

Dr. Dan N. Lantum, Area Medical Officer, Tiko Hospital: Letter to The Director of Education, Education Department, Buea, on 18th April, 1968: "This client of ours who is a worker of yours in the category of clerk in the Education Office, Kumba, has attended my hospital in frail health today. This is related to the fact of long strain without rest for about three years.

We are satisfied that he is medically unfit to carry on any work at the moment and will need a long leave of at least two months beginning forthwith. We are recommending therefore that necessary action regarding his leave emoluments and the usual Government requisites be rectified in his favour in the earliest opportunity. After his leave we will like to have the pleasure of examining him and advising you further about his health."

Dr. Schwarz, Acha-Tugi Hospital: Letter to The Medical Officer, Dr. Lantum, Tiko Hospital on 7th May, 1968: "We have seen your patient Benedict Tanka on 22/4, 29/4 and 7/5/68.

Diagnosis confirmed: Schizophrenia, paranoide. Other results: Hgb 87%. Microfilaria in skin-snips pos. Rohrschach Psychodiagnostic: not very pathological. Treatment administered: Personal interviews, and Psycholepticum per injectionem resulted into a relaxing sleeping-course during 1 week at home.

Subjectively he feels a bit better; main complaint is the sleeplessness. We advised him to postpone his plans with G. C. E. etc. Paranoid ideas now not openly admitted but referred to dreams. P. S. Patient deposited a notebook full of dreams; on request we could send it in."

Dr. Dan N. Lantum, Area Medical Officer, Tiko Hospital: Letter to The Director of Education, Buea, on 17th June, 1968: "I am happy to release Mr. Tanka now to you. He is now much improved and can resume work. But as he has great propensity for relapsing into his old condition, I am here recommending that he be removed from environments that are likely to precipitate his old condition. Bamenda and Buea are likely to constitute favourable environments for his health considering the physical and social climate. But wherever he resumes I would further recommend that he be put on light duty i. e. duty free of many intellectual challenges and exacting contemplation, for at least one month. "

Dr. Muna, Medical Officer, Mazam Division, General Hospital, Bamenda: Letter to The Senior Education Officer, Bamenda, on 4th November, 1969: " We have been following Mr. Tanka medically since August 22nd 1969 and have now noted considerable improvement in his condition. I recommend that he should return to work, be placed on light duty that does not require exactness and too much concentration, and be observed for 3 months. I cannot rule out the possibility of a relapse in this case. Buea now appears to be an untried but possibly favourable environment for him to work. Thank you. "

Dr. Schwarz, Acha-Tugi Hospital: Letter to The Medical Officer, Dr. Lantum, Tiko Hospital on 16th Dec., 1968: "I consider Mr. B. N. Tanka bodily fit to undergo the training course without physical exercises and farmer work and sports. Mental difficulties are likely to occur. "

Dr. J. L. Ngu, Specialist Internist, General Hospital, Victoria: Letter to Professor A. Boroffka, Dept. of Neuro-Psychiatry, University Hospital, Ibadan, on 18th June, 1971: "Mr. Tanka Benedict has been under my care as an out patient since his return from Ibadan.

I am pleased to report that the satisfactory progress he made whilst under your care has been maintained since his return to Cameroons. He does, however, have episodic attacks bordering on fugue, and occasionally has dreams similar to those he related to you prior to therapy. Furthermore we have investigated his periodic attacks of "pain in the small of the back" and retrosternally, and we have been unable to find any organic cause or causes for these. I am therefore recommending to the Director of Medical Services that Mr. Tanka keeps his follow-up appointment with you scheduled for August this year. His current therapy comprises chlordiazepoxide, Benzhexol, stelazine and chlorpromazine hydrochloride in the doses you recommended, as my initial attempt to gradually reduce the dosage of these aggravated his symptoms. "

4. WRITINGS BY BENEDICT NTA TANKA

PART I: DISEASES AND WITCHCRAFT IN OUR SOCIETY: COMMENTARY

In writing this story I have made mention of some names. Some of which are names of persons still living or dead and the rest are names which I knew when the incidence occured. As this is a story which may be teaching to each and every one of us, I plead to those whose names appear in this story from time to time not to be upset.

It is a common thing in our society that man suffers partly from God-sent disease and partly from disease that spring up as a consequence of man's wickedness to other human lives. While science is fast in diminishing some of our very common diseases, more artificial ones creep in through human disregard to his brother.

There is nothing doubting and people well versed in the occult sciences will tell you that witchcraft does exist. I have never believed that there is something like that, but I was forced by a supernatural occurence to believe that there exist Witchcraft.

A boy who was born wholesome was bewitched and he became impotent. One of his hands was paralysed and the disease was in him for four years. The hand was dead. He felt no pain even at the application of an electric current. No hospital could treat it. This same child was taken to a herbalist and in two days he was well. He was able to play. His hands were powerful again. When questioned, the herbalist said the child was poisoned and that no medical Doctor would cure him except a Witch Doctor.

If Witchcraft exists, does it exist in all societies? Is it a disease by itself? It whould be a disease by itself if its aim is to disable a person or take away life for selfish aims. All diseases are well known in a European society and can easily be eradicated by Doctors as they are the men of Science. All such things like operation, invention of the Submarine, the Air planes and all what not, I call them a Witchcraft to the European Community because it is a means, to improve man's standard of living with his neighbour or neighbouring countries. The Question still suspends, of what use is Witchcraft to an African Community? Is it not for jealousy: for personal agrandizement and for his lack of respect for God's Creation?

There are various diseases that spring up as a result of this in most African Societies and many die for this contribution. Such diseases are elephantiasis, swollen stomach, Blindness, Madness and Deafness just to mention a few.

I am writing this in a Cameroon society which is still underdeveloped in medical fields. This poses a lot of difficulties to the Engineers of this field. Usually, much medicine, time and energy is wasted to attend to such cases presented by human inferiority over their neighbours' lives. In very rare cases a few may be treated. Such diseases are hard sometime to be treated by international specialists. What then is witchcraft to our society? It is not a development but a lowering of man's standard. It should not be surprising for one to hear that men undergo courses in Witchcraft and graduate and become pests to human life. Its purpose is for envy and for loss of lives only.

One may think that I am just biassed with the society or that I am singling out myself from such a group, but as there is no smoke without fire, I am quoting an example in the next paragraphs that follow. Something interesting happened to me similar to what I have been saying in the above pages. It is right now still without solution, still strange but its effects have had far reaching and disastrous torments on me especially my brain, my alimentary canal, my chest both internally and externally, pains all over my whole body. It is something real, something worth knowing, something mysterious that occured to one man in a Cameroon society. I am writing to know from my readers what it meant. It has cost me time, energy and money before I am able to think a little. I have roamed round the federated state of West Cameroon, for this. I have received treatment from many hospitals and from some herbalists. My actions as a result of the illness were singled out by internal and state provocation but nonetheless the whole issue is still confounding and irrational. If there is no smoke without fire whosoever has consented himself/herself to this should imagine to have carried the burden ladened by this and see how far he would go.

The episode below is a full account of what happened to me. I am writing this in the North but the scene of the mystery is centred around Kumba in the federated State of West Cameroon. Although this illness which I may call it a plague of Cameroon Modern society afflicted my memory, it should be known to every-one that every statement made here is a fact, and original.

Events leading up to the scene:

It was 19th of March, 1968. I was sleeping in my bedroom. I felt some pains in my right toe. Sleepy as I was I recognised some figures by the side of my bed. They were shadowy figures of Mr. Andela and Doctor Lantum. The Doctor's figure was faint because he stood behind Mr. Andela. Prior to this, I had felt a heart-beat movement through my body and I heard a voice in my body saying, "I am Mr. Andela;[1] Secretary to the Prime Minister. Do not speak to me. I will speak to you". This movement was very unusual and faster than the pulse of the heart. It made my heart beat faster than before. I got up from bed and walked up to my table, pulled out a book from my Library and tried to read it. I couldn't just glance through it as I was fatigued by the activities of the day. I got a piece of paper and was making a shopping list.

I heard and felt a piercing sound pricking through my head into my skull from Mr. Andela. Then followed a command from the same person that I should be very careful with myself. A few moments later as I sat stupiffied and dumbfounded, I heard another voice from the Prime Minister. The Prime Minister said, "Walk to the door, stand on your heels and look to the left and right and you will see a girl whose name is Angela Ndefru [2] by the left hand-side near your window." The sounds came from my house but the persons were invisible. However, though in such a trance, I shuffled to the door with the heart beating with fright. I performed the action but no person was seen nor even a voice heard from around but the moonlight was blazing around the whole compound. It was a miracle. My heart was almost going away. It was just about eight o'clock but there was dead silence in the whole vicinity.

I took courage and continued my shopping list for the following morning. The sound grew louder and more severe on my head. The sound was penetrating through the pores on my head and through a depression, which its violent effects have caused on my head into my brain. Sooner or later many voices were heard telling me to write this and that. Was this a group of ruffians, a miracle, or a dream? If it was a dream, why should I be up? Despite the confusing voices, I made my shopping list at my will.

The next day which was the 21st of March was to be my feast day. My thoughts were centred round my christian birthday. I got my missal and read the life history of St. Benedict. All this I did in opposition to the mysterious voices.

My Christian Birthday:

But what happened on the 21st of March 1968? I gave no money for shopping to my brother nor did I make mention of it to him, otherwise he should have reminded me of it.

At 5 a.m. on this day, I woke up from sleep and had myself ready for the church. As I was leaving the house, the voices of the previous evening came back again. The same voice of Mr. Andela commanded me to buy the following things: - a small bottle of Guineas stout, a bottle of grenadin, two yellow loaves of bread and a tin of margerine. It was a common place that each person who spoke to me introduced himself/herself. For example "I am Mr. Andela, speaking to you." I was led from the house by him and half way gone another person in the name of Lonka A took over and led me right to the church. She was all the time advising me and telling me that I can't write good English. As the voice continued, she said she was speaking right from Mankon and was also going to the church. The voice of Lonka said that they were many and were able to see me because their eyes were opened but for myself, I was still a child.

Inside the Church:

Right inside the church as I was kneeling down, I was taught by voices even if I was doing the right thing, how to say my prayers and how to genuflect. Those who advised me were Mr. Andela, Rose who termed herself to be Lonka A [3], Mr. Ako and Mr. Gabriel Tanke [4]. No one can imagine my attitude during this time but myself. I was so pricked in heart by an unearthly sensation, so irritated and nervous that my prayers were not properly recited. I was made to start learning afresh like an infant. What It meant to the mob that was so concerned, I do not know. But everything as it stands reflects onto the originator, be he spirit or a human being. In the above passage the facts are original and occured to the person during the day (not in a dream). But in Buea he had a dream where he saw Mrs. Atabong in a class-room cancelling his composition.

The Scene at the Market:

I made up straight for the market to buy what the unseen persons told me. No body knows how and why I had to obey commands from a pack of nuisances who might have taken different forms to torture a miserable soul. I bought those things where I was commanded to buy by the voices and in that madness the magerine was forgotten and only to be collected later.

The journey from the Market to the House:

The same voice of Mr. Andela said I was really in his command or rather that he has taken command of me for the day because I had obeyed him so much. He also led me back to the house this time. He urged me to get home and take the beer and provision and that he would inform the Educating officer about it and she would not do anything to me. Continuing, he told me so many people whom I could not see but that they were all seeing me and that I have large family of 163 persons [5] who were present at the time. Probably he meant a large family of friends. A few of the names he mentioned were Mr. Andela, Mr. Ako, Christine Fonten, Christopher Mohammed and Lonka A in the name of Rose, and Betty. He told me that they were all seeing me but as a child, he repeated, I couldn't see them. The whole of this scene was dominated by Mr. Andela who did all the talking and was very much in opposition to Lonka A who criticised my English. He Mr. Andela read out some sentences constructed by Lonka A and said that was no English. He deplored her criticism and admonished her not to compare her English with mine. He said it was a shame to her because she was merely reading out what was written by another person. After all this comparison and advice I got to the house at 8 a. m.

My Unwarranted Feast:

I acted as if I was in the military force. Everything was done by a command. I was in a world ruled by spirits. I sat down to my feast under the wings of the heavens or seraphines that had come to share with me on my feast day for better or for worse. As soon as it was ended I hurried back to the office. If it was the work of man, Great Kumba would have known the man. If the work of God no single soul in Kumba would know. But what does it mean to you if someone saw you on that day and said "you are now a man"? If it is the work of man;

what highlight does this event portray on the inhabitants of this locality? It may be a small occurence to you. Can it repeat itself some where? [6]

On the way to office:

The whole scene consisted of a series of advice. Some people telling me this, others that, and the event turned into confusion. "Do not follow the road to the hospital at night. Always go by the main road and let's see he who will give you a lift as many people say they know you," the voice of Mr. Andela said. At last I got to the office at 9 a.m. I was late for one and half hours.

Inside the office:

I signed the attendance register and went straight to my table. I took three letters to register and the voice of Lonka was severe on me. Lonka was so hot and did not want me to work. My head was heavy and was full of vibrating air which swept in with great force through my ears and the pores on my head.

After thirty minutes, I was not able to register one of the letters. I was weak, tired and my head was sweating. I went up to my boss who said he would not let me go until 2 p.m. I got back to my sit but was unable to persevere. Even the Chief of the office could not allow me go. He merely gave me a chick [7]. But I had to go home. There was no need sitting down in such an agony from mysterious voices. I left the office without a word and went home. The voices continued talking as I was going home. A girl rode past me on a Mobylete and one of the voices told me that the girl was a devil and that she had once been a girl friend to Mr. Andela. I was warned to be careful in dealing with people because some of them were devils.

At Home:

I went to bed and in the evening, I was sitting in the parlour. Mr. Tona came to my house that same evening for a visit. We had a short conversation with him but I was not able to entertain much talking. After a while, he bid me good night and off he went. I saw him off just at the door. Before Mr. Tona came in, Dr. Lantum had come to me in a form like that of a fly, walked across my head and in a while he was talking within me. The most striking thing about this is that the fly which was speaking, introduced itself to me to be Dr. Lantum. He told me to be very careful with myself and that I should fix my eyes always to a point when I am thinking of something evil. He told me not to speak so much to Mr. Tona who was speaking to me. As I was ill, I should not speak so much to him because my lungs will wear out. As the whole scene was dominated by no persons, invisible beings whose voices were heard came in, in their forms and advised me [8].

The three Ghosts:

As I laid in bed on my back sleeping, I felt a stream of cold air almost ladened with moisture coming through the window. A figure of a woman appeared almost naked. My hair stood on end and I shivered in bed. It climbed on my radio and walked across my head bed and then disappeared. I seemed to have recognised the figure, probably that of Christine Fontem [9].

An hour later, another came in and bounced three times on my stomach because I laid on my back. It was not heavy so that I felt no pains nor did I fear as with the first ghost. This too I recognised to be that of Betty [9].

Lastly the third ghost came in and laid down by my side in a well sewn skin of a snake. She played on the bed, beating her legs on the bed. I recognised this too but the ghost wasn't happy at all because of the skin and cried and struggled to remove it and in that struggle it fell down and went under the bed where it disappeared. This was Rose.

One may doubt this story but it is something as I said before that is original. It is not just a made up story to arouse public interest to sympathy or to show a keen mind of imagination. On the next day I made a thorough check up of my radio and found that it was bad.

The Doctor's Examination:

The next day I went to the District Medical Officer for consultation. I told him what had happened to me. He examined me and said there was nothing wrong with me at all; yet I was weak, helpless to myself and unable to go to work. He prescribed a few tablets for me. I took them and went back to the house.

The two Butterflies:

On returning from the hospital, I went straight to my bed. Dr. Lantum was in me as I laid gasping into space and contemplating on what to do. Soon a butterfly flew into my bed room and alighted onto my bed curtain. The Doctor told me the first Butterfly was Rose signifying love and that if I were yet a man I should be able to know what to do. A few minutes later a second Butterfly came in and flew past the first one and the Doctor remarked that it was one Vincent Abang who had come to shelter the first Butterfly, Rose, because it was tired.

The Laughter:

I sat down in the parlour bearing the pains patiently, still perplexed and did not know what to do. Happiness had disappeared and in a moment a light, yellow slender figure appeared directly in front of me. I recognised it immediately.

It was laughing gently and as soon as I recognised it, I was induced by the figure to laugh too. I was alone in the house but then I was not more alone because the picture was fresh in my memory. Another voice talking in me said the girl whose figure I had just seen would be teaching in the Buea Road R. C. M. School, Kumba during the holiday. Right from this scene onwards the figure, Rose by recognition, had by induction infused the laughing stock spirit into me [10]. It almost became a habit in me and later on it became an unconscious action. To many especially Mr. Elonge, and a few others they wondered because my behaviour was very unusual and some said I was mad.

A Reverend Father's advice:

A few days after my very Reverend Father, my Counsellor in a spiritual form pricked me to get the radio to the town for repairs as no person would come round to sympathise with me. I ordered my brother to go with me to the town with the radio. The fault in the radio was discovered and repaired. But it did not last long, just for a day. The Reverend Father asked me to go to Mr. Andela and tell him what has happened to me. This I did. I went right to Buea and met Mr. Andela in his office. I told him the course of events but he in reply said he did not understand what it meant. I went back to Kumba in bewilderment. It sounds ridiculous for me to be praising Spirits but then, the manner in which some of these voices spoke to me or advised me really showed me that some of the spirits liked me. Even if they were inflicting me with pains and loneliness, there may be something good in it, for "good are the uses of adversity, which like a toad, ugly and venemous; yet wears a precious jewel in his head. Find tongues in trees, sermons in stones and running brooks and good in everything. I will not change it". This quotation from Shakespeare encouraged me.

The White Board:

I opened my eyes when I heard a sharp piercing noise from the camp. I glanced through my bed curtain and suddenly a white Board appeared in my bedroom and the inscriptions "Queen Elizabeth II" were boldly written on it. Then after this the real figure of the Queen appeared in transparent apparel. It was so majestical, quite quiet, but distinct like coloured pictures and in a few moments it disappeared. There was no talking or advice from any spirits nor was there any voices from the vicinity. Every place was dead silent. What does this mean? I asked myself.

Myriads of Shadowy figures:

Right from the time of my illness, I made one chair a permanent seat. I would like to sit on that particular chair any time I was in the parlour. While I sat down in perplexed thoughts and was waiting for my fate, not even a soul came in. What must be wrong? Even the usual persons that come round at times for a visit? There must be something brewing around. But scorns followed after scorns from the Gendarme Camp. Some people said: Mua qua-qua forty, Mua qua-qua forty [11].

I guessed the voices and seemed to know the persons who were speaking. But if there were voices of persons I knew what did they want in the camp at that material moment? Voices of the three ghosts I had mentioned earlier. Was it imitation from some people? The mistakened identity in voices was a sure proof to me that some personalities were dramatising my actions [12]. But there was one heavy voice which was echoing [13] from time to time and it seemed to be that of a Gendarm who was probably questioning some girls and women.

In the midst of the happenings and the love catch words, I couldn't just say exactly to myself anything about the subterranean movement. All this time, I was lying in bed and when I suddenly fell asleep, I heard an angelic float [14] which sounded through my ears with soft and gentle melody that sent me to a deep sleep. After floating, the person changed to singing. The voice chanted like that of a white girl but as it was interrupted by laughter it seemed that it was Christine who was singing. The music blared so sweet in my ears that I suddenly burst into laughter and when I opened my eyes and looked up the ceiling, where the voice came, it was quite quiet [15].

I saw many frightful shadows. I was now really sitting down in the house when I saw these shadows. Each time I sah a shadow, I heard the man with a heavy voice from the Camp dictating and commanding. He was saying something pertaining to the shadow. The shadows were faint figures of persons which appeared and lasted for about a few seconds. Figures of frogs, snakes and birds were seen in the house. This was a terrible scene. I asked myself, were these the shadows of the voices that have been speaking to me?

Although those were to me like shadows, yet some spoke to me by wispering through my ears and some were really shouting. Others termed themselves to be devils: namely Demond Tipuan, Demon Aja, Demon Tashih and Demon Adu and so on [16]. There were many other devils who came in often and whenever I thought of something without voicing it out they would quickly say that I have been thinking about this and that [17]. Some of these spirits advised me to be very careful in Kumba. Demon Tipuan was such a funny personality. He spoke to me in shouts with a commanding voice, always shouting and dancing. Sometime he would plant his legs into the ground and disappeared and came out at another corner.

The Scene by the Window:

There was a bed covered with grass outside and I often heard voices from the Camp saying, "your grave is behind your house," I thought I would die as far as I could not understand what was happening to me. I believed these people who were talking in the vicinity knew more about my fate and that the said grave was a scorn to me before my death as many of them had already predicted that I was alone and no one would burry me when I died. They were really hooligans in their mode and it beats my imagination why uniformed officers should indulge themselves to torment a perplexed sick man. Why should their speech relate to what he was doing? These were the questions I asked myself and I concluded that they were consented.

It was not sooner when the disturbances from the vicinity were interrupted by a theatre of shadowy crowd which ranked from the least to the greatest man in the country. The humorous demon, Tipuan led the scene singing and shouting, danced from corner to corner. He would stand erect, plant his legs into the ground, disappear and shoot out at one end. I leaned against the window and noticed the shadow crowd which was motionless with the exception of Tipuan who attracted the attention of the crowd by his singing and movements.

He displayed my life history from infancy to the present moment and I could see myself going through the different stages of development. The time I started crawling, the time I began to speak and so on. This was so surprising to me especially when he said that he was asked by some people to invoke the different scenes of stages in my life. At this time, I noted two different things, namely invoking the dead and invoking the past actions of one's life. To my greatest amazement, I heard him calling the names of all my friends. Those with whom I have been at school and others I made after leaving school. A little while after Tipuan's exhibition of my life history, I sighted Betty moving forwards and looking straight at me. I have grown old to the scene that I laughed not for pleasure but for grief because there was no clue to what was actually happening. She raised up her hand and spoke some broken sentences in my native tongue, looked at me in a pretentious love scorn and vanished. I said to myself, what really does this convey of the characters of this story? I am still a child. Yes, they have said it but then how will I know that they want me to be like them when they present different forms and will not show me the clue to be like them? It still amazed me the more when I noticed the president of the Republic offering a present of sixteen thousand francs to someone. Everything was dramatized in perfect tranquility although interrupted by little noise at certain intervals. But after the offer or gift, distant voices from the concentration camp [18] echoed: "That is money for your Over sasse order." This touched my nerves and nobody will convince me that this was not human demonstration either for good or for worse.

I then thought of my order which I had made. Everything about my order had been settled and I was only waiting for the arrival of the material; for what else on earth is that demonstration for? As the sun glittered through the air, the crowd soon dispersed and I walked back into the parlour and sat down on my chair and my thoughts became more complicated. I sat down with severe head ache and supported my chin with my hand and leant on one side of the chair [19].

In the Parlour:

It was not long when I sat down gasping into space in front of me, quite perplexed and worried in mind at the chain of events that have happened but were still unknown to me. When I wiped my face, I saw a whole long Indian file came in by the back door. I saw many friends, some of my department, and others of different walks of life. As each person danced in he reminded me of some relationship between me and the person in life. I noticed a girl throwing some pictures onto the floor and a lady did same with some bananas. The crowd which danced in and singing in pidgin disappeared at the door leading to my bed room.

But was this an outward sign of pleasure or scorn shown in an indirect way? The persons I saw were all responsible persons. What on earth will make them present themselves in that manner? Was this day dreaming? No, it was not day dreaming because many instances had shown me right at Kumba, and whenever I went in the Republic that there is an underground movement behind me which remained hidden behind the curtain.

The Second Crowd:

I noticed two lawyers stepping in their official uniforms and reading very voluminous books. I knew two friends with whom we have been at school, Obiekwe and Nunyello and one person, the third was a school Mistress, Miss Susanah Uzo who had been my teacher in school in my early days in the primary school. This particular lady has appeared to me several times in my dreams and in one occasion, I pictured myself in a tribe in the Eastern Region of Nigeria and I was introduced to groups of persons some of whom I knew and some were just new acquaintances. The crowd entered in silence, only danced and gesticulated and the lawyers solemnly looked at their volumes, read in silence and in a while they vanished.

The Third Crowd:

The president of the Republic came out of my bedroom into the parlour. He was in a light, blue gown, and a small white cap. As soon as he came into the parlour, he raised up his hand to shake hand with me. I only guessed at the image. It was quite real and distinct. Tipuan like the demoniac guard sprang up from one corner and said that he was a demon. He told the president a short story in his life as a president. He told him that he, Tipuan has been coming to his residence. He also said that the president wanted to board a plane from Douala to some destination but he Tipuan got there and warned the president that there would be an accident on the route and that the president should not go. He later on asked the president whether he has forgotten his person and the third time he admonished him not to board the plane. The president said he had not forgotten. Tipuan asked the president whether he as the head of State can allow him come back to life again. The president said he was guarded by demons and that never in the history of revelation has anyone dead come back to life. As he altered [20] this, he waved his hand in the air indicating refusal to suggestion and smiled at the same time his hand was waving. The president facing the crowd of spirits remarked about my house. He said in many occasions he had been coming to my house for protection and he found the house a suitable quiet place. He had been watching me and had found no fault in me although he had heard from many about me. He had been coming in my house to know who I was, and upon his findings, he found me to be good. On saying this the ghosts all vanished to their kingdoms and Tipuan whose aim is to come back to life and teach the rest of the world what he has seen, went him under the house with his American girl and I saw a paradise. A well built house, gorgeously illuminated with a type of blue light which matched with the painting of the floor. It was well furnished and I saw a type of chicken which was not of this earth.

The Snakes:

I saw two coarse snake like figures lying on one arm of the chair directly opposite me. Those figures could take any form. As I kept on guessing, I noted their heads transforming into human heads and their hands vice versa. Their teeth were as white as snow. Their looks, laughter and actions portrayed that the snake girls were in love [21]. What did all this show me? Of course, it is just too obvious that my eyes were not yet opened for vision of the world around. As the voices had earlier told me that I was a child, all these meaningless scenes were definitely a sure proof to me that man lives in a diversity of ways and satan has great influence over him.

While the shadowy figures kept on guessing at me, two flies alighted onto my head. One walked from my head down to my left hand side and went off and it was the fly of Betty because it introduced itself to be Betty. The other pierced through my left handside and came out of my left leg, then walked down to my private part. This was the fly of Helen. These were the snake girls in the form of flies. Helen walked up and down around that area and would speak, advised, said this and that. I got angry because of much talking and unnecessary amusement from strange ghosts. Imagine it was almost a week now since the voices started and I had not known anything about them. The fly was offended at my reactions and flew off in annoyance.

The Embalmment:

I went out to the back door and heard from a voice such words like "telepathy", "opaque", and "embalmment". Another voice talked of people being on the same line. It continued by saying that I would be linked to all my friends and they would be speaking to me wherever they happened to be. Another one said the Prime Minister was on the highest line in the country and he was linked to other great men and countries. There was no need asking questions to me because right from the onset the events have been supernatural. I merely walked back to my seat to bear patiently the burden of the plague. It was a devilish plague.

To many, this may appear childish and somewhat false but it should not be taken to mean otherwise because it is something which is quite real and originally told by someone who was suffered innoncently to the amusement of the public at the time for either his betterness or misery in life.

The first fly went through my left handside and came out from my chest. I can remember two or three names that were introduced to me. The first one was Honourable Lafon, the second, Honourable Jua and the third Francis Shey, who told me that they had heard of my illness and had come to visit me but in a form which was different from mine. The first two also said they were embalming me, but it was so surprising to me if someone should be embalmed alife. I was told that about fifty-two different persons went through me at the moment and among them were my parents. My mother pricked through me from my left handside and came out of my left toe while my father went through my right handside and came out of my right toe.

The movement in me was so electrical that I imagined their movements in me and I pretended to be seeing them swimming in my blood vessels but each would say, don't look at me in that manner [22].

During this time, Father Sullivan was all the time on my head [23] and before any set of flies alighted onto my body he had already told me everything about them. My parents spoke grammar and vernacular and it was so distinct and they told me that in which form they could speak any tongue.

From the onset Hon. Jua found difficulty in going through my body and he went back to lead himself as he said and at the second attempt he pleaded and went through with no difficulty. Imagine the piercing through my veins and other blood vessels. Expanding my veins, and what do you expect from this? Loss of blood, increase of absorbing capacity by the blood vessels and a general weakness in the entire body, are sure results. The patient is made to drink much.

Acrobatic Scene in the evening:-

Against the wall five shadows of immense height appeared carrying stones on their heads. They were taking an exercise. They would sit down in crouching position with the stones standing on their heads at ease. They stretched their hands sideways, upwards and downwards, pulling in their muscles and one of them, Aja, told me that that was a way they used to develop their muscles in school. He told me that in those German days they were so good in school in athletic and football. He demonstrated how he used to play football and that in his days there was no youth in school or in his village that could withstand him. Then Aja went into a swimming pool and dived in with a snake and told me that I would be taught how to play with the snake in the same manner and that my backbone would be straightened on a bamboo when I would go home and after that I would grow taller again and in that same instance Doctor Lantum told me that three Doctors had gone into me and that they counted the number of bones in my vertebral column andfrom their findings they have discovered that my age should be twenty five. He asked me to declare my age in my new station. The three Doctors were Doctor Lantum, Doctor Nasa and Doctor Chinda. The instant the second Doctor on the list went into me, I felt a scraping movement along my vertebral column and around my waste and just below one end of my stomach [24]. I concluded that my reproductive organs were displaced because usually once a month or so reproductive cement [25], the sperm in the male is eliminated naturally and periodically. But the more often I felt pains around that area and my remaining for a long time without the elimination of the cement as mentioned above, I almost believed that there was somewhing wrong. After this, the five demons continued with their advice. Adu was fairly old, the elder of Aja and each one of them was six feet tall. It appeared to me that there is no more growth after death. When once you are young you will continue to remain young and once old you continue to be so. As I looked it appeared to me that Adu had had a magic long bamboo into him symetrically and was showing me how he could carry about three or more other people in his mystic form in time of danger. I guessed him as he flew up and down and changed into many other forms. The demons were graded according to their powers of transformation. They threw certain things on my body and at the same time, they fell on my body, blood shook in my veins on the spot. They said they were making me a man and that they died when I was still very young. The other three did not know me. But two said I was delivered before their death.

They told me that their speed is like that of lightning. That when they left me within a second, they would be in U.K. or America. They were continuously making such flights to our home, Victoria, U.K. and America. They told me that they had travelled to different parts of the world, and that they were advised at home by people to come and visit me because they heard that I was ill. They repeated by naming the names of all those people I knew at Kumba. Tipuan who probably was the first demon to be with me took the other five and said they were going to a friend of mine who was staying in the Prison camp. Tipuan told me of his former contact with the girl whom I knew before ever I was sent to Kumba. He told me that he asked the girl of my whereabouts and she said I was at Buea. Sometime he left a message for her to tell me. He told me not to be doubtful because it is (more) easy for women to deal with the dead spirits than men. He further told me how he appeared to the girl in a school dormitory and that I would be taught how to invoke when I would go to my new station. Continuing he said he was invoked by someone in that school and the girl he appeared to in a dream was someone whom I know. Tipuan would go to the parents of the girl, talked to them as he told me and in a while he would come back, sometime he would come round handling Christine with his hand and would talk to me and Christine would also speak in my native dialect and they all asked me to be very careful and kind to Lonka A because they have known more about my relationship with her. Aja too was some what fun of Betty and they would bring her image in front of me and I would picture Aja doing some steps with her.

Afterwards I saw my file with my name boldly written on it. They showed me the file and opened it and showed me everything therein written about me by my boss. I was in the world of dead spirits. Some-time I would see some very short images like those of the "Maquisedes" [26]. As the hours rolled by, I felt a movement under my legs from the floor. Tipuan was speaking under my legs. He warned me that I should leave the parlour with immediate effect because so many persons would be coming there for a meeting. I insisted and sat down. Another person dressed in white, a familiar picture that of a teacher who had taught me in the primary school. He died many years ago. He was a good friend to Tipuan when still alife. He also warned me to take time where I was living. He showed on the blackboard how he used to teach me. He told me my scores in his examinations, my name and everything he knew about me before he died. They told me they knew all what was happening with me, my examinations and certificates. One of them told me that my school certificate was issued to someone else instead of me and that some certificates which I had in the G. C. E. Examination were also given to another person and that these people were all abroad studying. But continuing they said it had never been brought to my notice that I was successful in the examinations. I was given the reverse information. They made mentioned of some of the names. However, I did not believe it and not sooner after this, I saw the Principal of Sasse dressed in White. He was with one of my relatives who works there. He showed me eight hard oblong papers and said they were certificates in question and that they would be given to Betty to bring them that same evening. Betty would come to my house that same evening with Rose as well as everything of mine, book or so that got missing, or that was given out on loan and was not returned to me yet. As the voices continued they told me that some people who posses the snake [27] were getting information from my house from written documents even those that were locked up in the box. In the same manner my thoughts were read.

Identity in Voices:

At the same time, I heard someone spoke on the main road like Betty and later a much dignified and gentle heavy voice followed like that of Rose. I began to be convinced. I felt a flush of cool air rushed across my face and my nerves were stimulated to feel quite at home. I said I was going to get the result of that was going on or happening if the information given about the two girls' arrival and if the voices should not be a mistakened identity of the real persons presented by some irresponsible persons. By then I had taken my radio to the town and there was no source of amusement to a sick person who was probably an experimental tool [28] to some scientists or a political tool to some politicians or a miserable soul who was made to bear a yoke for the common good of the public interest. So I was somewhat a little bit pleased because I was told that the radio would be brought by those persons who were perhaps the only friends of mine specially allowed to come to me. A car glided slowly along the road, one of the flies on my head told me the car was conveying those my things and the girls. The car came to a stop and I was told it was the car of

Mr. Fish, the Manager of the B.I.C.I.C. Bank, Kumba Branch. I opened the door with anxiety and great expectation, obeying spirits. After all, all had deserted me and it was only the spirits that came in to advise me although I was sometime annoyed, it was because I am not a spirit myself hence I could not understand their purpose and I thought those girls would come and explain everything to me because I had seen their images and had been with them in my dreams. The door was ajar for the persons to walk into the house. As I looked, the lights of the car were not on. People were murmuring in the car. It started off again, after a few yards it rolled back again. I stood at the door to see exactly what was happening but the moonlight was so faint that I went back to the house. I was in the parlour waiting in vain for anyone to come. However, I did not lock the back door because I was told to leave it open for the visitors. I slept for sometime and when I raised up my head, I heard the foot-steps of someone who moved fastly past the back door to the hedge near the Kitchen and there I heard a sound as though something was thrown down. When everything was still, I crept out slowly and found nothing. I left the door open and went to bed.

In the night, I saw someone dressed like a Jew [29]. Tipuan was often by the window of my bed room. He would speak through my ear whispering and told me what was happening. The Jew was St. Jude [30] to whom I have been praying for help in my difficulties. He spoke to me saying that he has been hearing my prayers and that I should continue to pray. He told me when he was alife he used to spend all his time praying and he was so sociable whenever he went.

He said they in their own world also have politicians, different countries, and also carry on their own administration. Adding, he said persons can only see God through application and after doing their penances. He said God is kind and excuses those who died pegans and Tipuan told me that he has already crossed so many gates and he would soon see God. St. Jude walked up and down the small corridor which separated my bed with the wall. He said he has been in this world and still yet he likes to come out and enjoy himself and that he was out for justice and will not like to be suffered nor want someone to be suffered innoncently. His main object had been justice when he was alive and right up till now as a Saint he was strongly against those who were unjust. He walked up to my head bed and said he was leaving me.

I fell asleep again and when I got up, the lamp was still shining and no one had come in. No visitors. The voices had died a natural death. Who was my guard? Always by my window, Tipuan would speak and told me everything that was at home. How didhe come to know the girl, I love very much. How does he know all my friends and where they stay? This was what made me believe that Spirits have been talking to me. He talked of charms and that Father John [31] who had come to me and slept with me in the bed in his spirit would give me a charm which he left with him. Whenever he came round with a very powerful charm, my hair stood on end. Other members of our family who passed out of this world were with him and they had the ability to trap information from my thoughts [32]. They told me that it was easily got through the pulse of my heart. I could not say anything more but only concluded that the gospels have said it. There is nothing hidden under heaven [33].

The Cartoon [33a] of Heinekins:

The next day came and nobody came round nor was there any trace of someone who had come round when I had gone to bed. I asked of the friend I was expecting and was told that the friend did not come down for holidays. Similarly there was no trace that Betty had been around.

I sat me down in the usual chair panic striken with pressure of pain, I heard another voice on my head: "I am Sister Aquinas, principal of Queen of the Holy Rosary College Okoyong." She further told me that she is incharge of all the Catholic girls secondary schools in West Cameroon. She asked me to be very careful with myself. Then she made mention of a certain Rose in our Lady of Lourdes secondary school in Bamenda, in Mankon. She ordered me to buy a cartoon of Heinekins as my father would be coming to visit me. She admonished me not to feel lonely because I was not alone in the house. After some deep thoughts, I sent my brother for the beer. All what have been happening to me convinced me and I thought that my parents might come round, hence I bought the beer. She mentioned so many names to me and told me that some of the persons named would like to stay with me. She said that she would teach me English and later on I must teach in her school. She also made mention of one Conny Van Zanten who would like to stay with me and would teach me dancing and how to swim with the snake.

Later on two other Reverend Sisters came in. They were Sister Antonia and Sister Praidaig, Principal of girl's training Centre Fiango, Kumba. As soon as the beer was brought, the Reverend Sister Aquinas asked me to get a bottle and drink. What could I do other than obeying the Reverend Sister who spoke like an Angel and under whose administration my would-be Rose would come. She was often on my head and told me that she was getting information about what was happening in Kumba and would tell me later. She also told me a small story about the clock. She said the clock can speak to me. She showed me an example.

Sister Antonia came in and asked me to get my clock. I got my clock and kept it on the table. She told me she would enter the clock and speak to me. She asked me to pay attention and hear exactly her speech when the clock is ticking. This was done to my greatest amazement. One thing noteworthy was that I should keep the clock by my head bed to be speaking to me as a patient.

A few hours later, Sister Braidaig came and spoke to me and furnished me with information of what was happening. I was so sleepy and paid less attention and she asked me to go bed. While I was sleeping, she was quite quiet on my head in her spiritual form and on imagining what she must have been doing on my head. I guessed that she was probably knitting. She told me she was well armed and dangerous to anyone who proved daring. She said any person who ventured to come round for evil, she would be stern on him. It was just a few seconds when I heard her speaking angrily to an agressor who was not happy to see her on my head. She flew off from my head and turned out the man for goods. She came back and told me it was Mr. Elonge. She remained on my head for a long time till evening.

The Helicopter and the arrival of my Father:

It sounded doubtfully to me when a voice suddenly said that an helicopter was flown from Victoria to my home to convey my father and my sisters. If I were to argue this out, I would argue alone because there was no person to reason with me and the ghosts which told me were not visible beings to ask them questions. As I looked on, I saw four shadows of my sisters and another voice told me that they had come but were in the prisons barracks. I also learnt that my father had been there but was taken to Victoria by one Mr. Lawson of B. I. C. I. C., Victoria. The spirit further told me that my father came with some money for my girl, quite a fat sume of money for her dowry and that it might be misplaced. I feared this very much because I thought that he might take much drink and someone could even get it from him. It surprised me why he should go to Victoria without coming to me. If my father and sisters came they would have first of all come to me before going elsewhere particularly if they were aware of my ill-health. I was not convinced at all but the usual devils convinced me. Yet all the same, the poor man did not come at all. It was just an attempt for spirits to deceive me. Probably these were men in transformed appearances. Apart from my father and sisters the voices also told me that my three brothers had heard of what was done to me in Kumba and they came trekking to fight for this cause. When they came to the town, they were engaged in a snake and kneel fight. They also came to my house in the shadowy form and spoke to me. Another voice told me that my small brother with whom I was staying had been given the snake so that he used to see me everywhere I went in Kumba although I did not know. There was an instance when I really heard the movement of feet outside the house as though two people were fighting. One of those voices told me that it was Philip who was being interrogated in the snake form by one of my brothers. All this sounded stupid and very misleading to my mind. It was just an attempt by a set of persons to confuse whosoever was ill and to increase his ill-health.

The Spirit of Lonka A:

How the name Lonka originated is not known by even those who have been calling this name. Lonka is no person's name nor is it a nickname: But seeing that this is an age of incredibility, and epoch of foolery some men have been using this name to inspire their very low spirits. The name Lonka is only known by the writer of this story and by Betty and Rose. Any person who claims to know it may not interpret it in the proper way. Later on the writer of this story graded Lonka. So actually the writer knows only of two Lonkas and they have been fighting to wind more in their group.

As I sat down drinking some beer, I felt a crawling moment in my chest. Something was moving in like worm and piercing it, if I tried to stop the movement. Someone told me that it was the spirit of Lonka A. Lonka A was trying to see if I would bear the burden. Her spirit used to come to stay with me. It usually stayed with me for about two hours and one of the voices probably the reverend sister said that I was calm for her and I could shelter her for a longer period than the other person whom Lanka A was also putting to the test. Lonka's spirit also lived with Mr. Maimo; I was told this by some of the spirits. Her spirit used to enter me through my left handside and would go out through my right handside. I was told that her spirit could be with mine for a much longer period. At the same time my father's spirit also came to me and was with me for a whole day and it went out together with that of Lonka and when my right eye winked, I noticed something like a white cloud going out through my right eye into heaven. So the spirit of Lonka A was tested in me and I bore the burden.

Father Sullivan was on leave at this time, that is to say he was out of the Cameroon. Despite this, he told me he has been seeing me in his dreams and has also seen that I was ill and so he came round to be with me. To be with someone is an English expression which means a lot. He explained to me. To be with somebody is the same as to stay with him for an appreciable length of time in a visible manner whereas in another sense the person may be with or stay with you in an invisible form. He however, asked me to be careful when someone tells me that.

The Snap Shot by the Londoners:

As soon as the Reverend Father and his two English friends arrived the Father alighted onto my head and in his usual form he spoke to me. He informed me that he has come along with two friends but he would not disclose their names to me. Three of them would go into me and find out what was troubling me. He asked me to have on my night gown and then get a bottle of beer and set down on the table. He told me that his friends would snap me as soon as they came out of me. The two friends said nothing until everything they scheduled to do that evening was completed. I started drinking the beer and Father Sullivan told me that they were going to drink with me but in a way I would not notice it. As soon as they came out, they set their magic cameras and snapped me while I was drinking. When I stopped drinking a second snap shot was taken. The light suddenly went under the table and pierced through the centre of the table and at the same time they were examining me to see if there was any thing in me because there were rummours about that. After their examination, they said there was nothing.

I had earlier mentioned the time when Tipuan and his group threw some medicine onto my body and said that they were making me opaque and to find out what was in me. So this incidence was similar to it. The Father told me that he was getting offended as Rose failed to turn up and that he and Tipuan have in many occasions been with the parents and they would say one thing and then the other. At this juncture, they started talking about "Witch Money" which was given to the mission at Kumba to preserve. He said distance has made the money to be sent in that way and that was the shortest means of transacting business with distant tribes or countries. This sounded strange to my ears. The Father, as he went on told me that I should have no fear and that he has so many friends in Kumba who have been his pupils and now were holding responsible posts and some of the friends were those he made in social circles as Christians and in ordinary everyday life. As he said this he bid me goodbye and promised to be back the next day with Bridget Awasum and Rose Gana from London. He told me that Bridget was doing nursing in a town in Britain called Oxwald and Rose was studying medicine in London proper. When I referred Oxwald in my Atlas I did not find it.

The next day came and in the morning hours, Tipuan came in in a beautiful coat singing and with his American girl. He danced with the girl, spoke some English and my native tongue. The girl spoke some broken dialect and remarked that she liked me very much. When I went to the table for meal, she even came round and showed me how she would handle her cutlery at meal time but I paid no heed. As I was having a meal, I would notice them at one corner having the same meal with me. Then Tipuan told me that now I should know that whatever thing, I do eat or drink in that house, I am not doing so alone. It stroke my heart once more again because the people in the neighbourhood were speaking some broken Menka expressions, really very immoral; only a few of them were good to the ear. This gave me much food for thought. I thought that the figures which I had so seen and the voices heard together with other occurences were an artful trick played by some personalities to suffer me for their own selfish aims.

What was the point in these series of events without even a soul around to cool one's mind from various thoughts? The different forms, shapes and apearances of persons were done by the people of the locality to exhibit their sprituallism over other human beings. Some people must have transformed themselves into such figures especially figures of those people related to me either by family or friendly ties. It was an attempt to make me suspicious with anyone wherever I go. If there were any dead spirits like demons, the people must have invoked them either to frighten me or to tell them more about my mother's and father's families and my friends.

Bridget, Reverend Father Sulliven and Rose Gana came in and went into me and as each one of them swam through me he/she advised me to keep calm and be at home. As Bridget moved through me she said she would write to me in six months time when I am in Bamenda. She also said she would tell me a message in a letter and I would go to a hilly village to deliver the message. She snapped me and spoke to me that I should not be surprised to see them in that form because people everywhere live in that form. One will doubt why there was a mass of pricking or piercing through my body. For one, I will guess that, that was a mark of friendship, that is to say that the only way those people thought of showing their friendliness was to go through my body.

Formerly at the beginning of this story, Doctor Lantum advised me to read a section about Blood on a small pamphlet which was sent to me by the Eye Hospital, Kano. This was a prayer which he found it useful to me at that material movement because of the Mass of Piercing by people in their peculiar forms through me. That is to say Blood goes for nothing and it meant much to anyone who might have had evil aims towards that drama of spiritualism.

The two girls and the Reverend Father bid goodbye to me and went away. After an hour later they returned and Father Sullivan told me that there was some disturbances on the way by some Cameroonians and since he did not want to leave these girls, he had to come back with them to get some medicine from some English people in Kumba before leaving finally the next day.

The Speech:

At night and all of a sudden I pictured someone swimming above me by the side of the wall in a horrizontal manner as though his legs and hands were fixed to a spot so that he could push himself to any direction with ease. It seemed to me as if he had fitted himself in a sort of elastic skin which was fixed in position by air pressure. He started speaking in my vernacula and I quickly distinguished the person from the lot by his voice. He spoke rythmically as he swam in the air. His speech was on visits. He further said that he was heard everywhere in the town and that people were surprised to hear that tongue because they had never believed that that tribe had its own dialect and customs. He told me that they had been to many places in the Federated State of West Cameroon. Continuing, he said they were also going to speak to the Prime Minister only in their vernacula.

There were other small sized shadowy figures which could magnify themselves at will. Some would look at me, some would doubt me and others would recognise me. The person who spoke did so without a break for over thirty minutes. They made mention of "Nyamgzah" by which means those people can go to any place and they told me it was a witchcraft by which they had several encounters on the road with the Kumba people. In that witchcraft they can speak any language.

This came to a reality when in that state of confusion there was a war fare at the back door of my house. Elonge fighting with my father, Elonge being guarded by girraffs, Elonge shooting out a long tooth from his mouth [34]. My father changed into many forms viz, the snake, the snake pouring out fire from its mouth, the snake defending itself with shields and so on. Then in that struggle came Mr. Tandu to aid my father who was building a rocky house to protect himself.

The Doctor and the Soldier:

It was not long after the speech when in my same position I noticed Doctor Lantum's shadow entering through the front door which was locked. He moved smartly in and in a second he assumed the position and shape of the persons who had formerly given a speech. What did this signify? It meant that what or the form those people took was nothing or to be more exact, that I should not regard that as the highest witchcraft. That was the interpretation I gave to it. In the neighbouring room of the block in which I was staying there was a soldier, a friend to one of my co-workers. As I sat down watching the actions of the Doctor, the soldier's shadow pierced through the separating wall and sat directly in front of me on the table. It was quite calm but altered [20] no word. In a while the two shadows vanished.

The Warning and Maggot Movement:

I was now a spectacle of amusement to nobody but to spirits and probably to those who initiated the cool war [35]. I felt movements and heard speeches under my legs. Air was forced through my feet into my body and at the same time the voices above were forcing air into me through my ears and other air spaces on my head. The result was suffocation. Tipuan shouted and warned me to leave that parlour and go to my bed room and that I should leave the entire house the next day and go somewhere. After contemplating for about thirty minutes, I left and went to bed, I had been sleeping for a long time when I suddenly felt a movement in my matress like the streaming movement of maggots. All over my bed, in my pillows I was totally disturbed. I couldn't sleep. It was people moving in different forms. I heard Conny [36] speaking to me and moving in the manner described above. She talked of my going to Bamenda on transfer, my going to stay with her to do dancing and to learn more from her. She talked of Rose in whose school she teaches Domestic Science. She told me that she would be in London with me and she would be teaching me some Dutch and she and me would be studying at the London Hospital.

It should be noted that Tipuan was by the window and was all the time whispering through my ears and many other friends were doing same with the result that I was forced to listen either to one person or to none at all. The aim of so many people talking to me on different topics was merely to confuse me. Why? Because every average man knows that a single man cannot comprehend from about fifty persons at the same time. But fifty persons went into me to advise me in a second.

The Send off:

In the open air at the back of the house were two girls and two people dancing merrily and gaily although one of them was afflicted with pain; yet he pictured himself dancing with Betty outside while Kitts was stepping round with Rose.

The Flight:

Sooner after much merry-making and after Adhidjo's spiritual visit, the plane landed and only took one of them who was ill and it was arranged that Rose would follow later. Off he went waving gaily to the other three and he reached a certain hotel en route where he took enough for himself. He offered a bottle of beer to one of the waitresses but she turned down the offer. At Oxwald, Bridget, Rose and Reverend Father Sullivan's sisters, were waiting for Father Sullivan. In the long run he arrived and they were happy to get him in their midst. We stayed at Oxwald for three hours. Here Father Sullivan introduced me to his sister and advised her to be writing to me and to be visiting me whenever she is in London. He also told me that Conny from Holland would be here too in London and would like to be with me and to teach me Dutch.

After three hours, I bid goodbye to them at Oxwald and we left with Gana Rose whose father had given me ten thousand francs for her when I was leaving for London. She accepted to put me through Biology and Chemistry. I was soon introduced to my Chemistry teacher and also to my Biology teacher.

From the onset my lessons in Chemistry were very good but as I went further it became difficult and I was often encouraged by my teacher to create an interest in it.

Presentations:

Dr. Endely and Vincent Tanka appeared to me in bed while I was sleeping and handed a suit to me. I looked at it and did not know what to do. I stretched my hand, and the two shadows disappeared.

Dr. Chinda also came in and went through my left toe and advised me to be firm and not to mind what people thought about me.

The journey to Tiko:

Formerly, Tipuan and Conny had warned me to leave the house for sometime. The day had just dawned and another fly in the name of Mathias Ntah who said he was delegated by Father Sullivan to speak to me. He asked me to get some money and go down to Dr. Lantum who was living at Tiko. I saw no necessity of remaining there at Kumba without someone to treat me. I went to B.I.C.I.C. Bank to look for some money. While at the bank another fly which introduced itself to be Doctor Lantum told me that I would get him at Tiko in his house.

With the few francs, I caught a taxi. As I was riding the taxi, I had an unearthly experience. People speaking or whispering through my ears, I felt some undulating movement on the seat I was sitting. It appeared I was sitting on maggots or worms. I was shown a picture in front of the taxi, the picture of the Doctor, I was going to see. I call it unearthly because when I got to his house I saw the same picture [37], the same posture, size and colour but I burried everything in my mind. It was yet still a miracle. Who can explain?

I got to his house when he was still at work but his wife asked me to wait for him. A few seconds later, he came in and I greeted him. He took his seat near his wife and I was drinking some beer which his wife had offered me. I introduced myself to him and told him the object of my mission. As I said this, he looked straight into my eyes but I continued to say much about him especially when I mentioned that he had been my teacher sometime and that he has only forgotten me. On hearing what was wrong with me, he asked me to come the next day.

I went up to Mutengene and the next day I came down, confused by the many voices and fatigued by much pain, my wrist watch dropped in the vehicle I boarded and that was the end of it. There was no way of getting back that golden and durable watch. It had gone to one who had not laboured for it. Even though I could recollect the image of the driver very well in my memory, it was no more my watch. The landrover by which I had come had dropped me and passed down to the market but as I stood thinking, the driver rode swiftly past me, though looking at me refused to stop when I tried to stop him.

Anyway, something else new had created more room for thoughts but I must see the Doctor. It is really from this juncture that I believed that some of those voices were misleading [38]. One of the spirits in me said that I should go and that the Doctor would give the watch to me. I went to the hospital, paid the consultation fee and met the Doctor. He took note of my complaints and prescribed some medicine for me. This was a different Doctor, a lady Doctor, Dr. Martins. Dr. Lantum, the Senior Medical Officer was in his office. After my examination and treatment, I went to the Doctor in question. He looked at me with great pity and prescribed more medicine for me. Then he took his pen and wrote three letters. Viz one to the Director of Education requesting him to grant me a two months sick leave, one to the Education Officer, Kumba, and the other to the Medical Officer, Acha Tugi telling him to give special attention to me and to give him a medical report after he has released me. I took all the three letters. I went firstly to the Director of Education and delivered his own letter; then I went next to Kumba and delivered the other one to the Education Officer. The next day I packed all my things.

The Result of the Warning by Conny and Tipuan:

While I was away for two days at Tiko a snake had beaten the daughter of my neighbour, a Domestic Science Teacher with whom we were sharing the same block. The girl was taken to the Hospital and she died immediately. On my return I was told this. I was surprised. Then I quickly remembered what had happened to me. My little brother was not in the house. He had gone with that lady to the town because he was afraid to be in the house alone.

The next day he came and told me what happened to them. Then I remembered that sometime before I went to Tiko I felt something crawling under my bed and I felt something very sharp piercing the matress and pinning me. Then one of those mysterious voices was telling me something about the snake of someone who had died. The voice said that the snake was invoked right from afar, from my place. This was not a reality to me because I do not think that dead men have snakes [39]. Once a person is dead everything about him finishes. What was all the talking about? The voice said the snake was under my bed and it was loving me. The next morning, I saw some dark figure under the bed. I asked my brother to find out what it was. On his findings he told me there was nothing. This happened before I went to Tiko but I only brought this to memory after my neighbour's daughter was killed by a snake; then I believed that the voices were right, although I did not take them serious.

I told my brother to pack everything immediately. I did not want to leave him in that house alone. We arranged everything in the house in proper order. I asked him to pack everything of his and when he was ready we left for Bamenda. The following day, I sent him to Widekum and passed to Acha Tugi and delivered the letter to the Doctor, a tall, simple gentleman who on looking at the letter recognised the Doctor who wrote it.

He asked me to go to the waiting room for a test. I went there. He came and gave me only pictures to be looking at. After he had left me his wife came and conducted the test. After finding out the final results, he admitted me as an out patient. For three weeks I received treatment. More of the voices were still troubling me all the time. During the day, during the night and at every blessed second. In fact it was almost becoming a nuisance and it was really then that I could not bear the pains. Some of the spirits say:- "It is very easy for the thread of a camel to go through the eye of a needle than for a rich man to enter the kingdom of heaven" [40]. This was not from voices of men but from the fly that was suspending on my head. It was common too because people were also trying to amuse themselves with what they knew about my illness. They were making the same sounds as those I had heard on my way to Tiko, in Tiko and in Kumba. From this I believed that it was a planned act.

The Doctor's Report:

After three weeks, the rate at which my heart was beating reduced. The dizziness in my head and pains were relieving [41] me gradually. The Medical Officer of Acha, Dr. Schwarz wrote a report about my health and gave me to give to Doctor Lantum.

The visit to my Parents:

As soon as I finished with medical attention, I went home to report to my parents because the news was erroneously told to them. Everyone of them believed that I was mad and that I was moving from place to place with little knowledge of what I was doing.

Before I went most people had told me that my parents knew what was wrong when I narrated the course of events to them. As I was in a hurry my father only told me to go and return later for proper investigation and treatment. Within three days, I left and went to Kumba.

Return journey to Kumba:

Although still weary, I went back to my station leaving Philip behind because schools have started while I was still on sick leave. However, I had arranged that he should go to a new school. After a night at Okoyong, I boarded a vehicle and got to Kumba in good time.

As soon as I got to the house everything was in chaos. Rats spoiled everything in the house. This added more pains to my health.

Report to Dr. Lantum:

The next day I went to Tiko after I had done some little bit of tidiness in the house and exchanged words with a few persons. I met the Doctor in his Office and gave him a letter from the medical officer, Acha Tugi. He read it and asked me if there was any improvement. I told him the tension was not as great as before.

All the same, he prescribed more medicine for me and advised me to buy medicine from the chemists whenever I am worried by the symptoms of my illness. He also advised me to report to Tiko too when there are any signs of the illness coming back to me again.

After examining me, he wrote and recommended for my immediate transfer either to Bamenda or to Buea because from his observations he found that I was affected by the social and physical climate of Kumba. He also wrote and recommended that I should be prohibited from all intellectual challenges and exacting contemplation. I went to the Director of Education and presented the letter to him but he delayed the transfer and this had a great effect on my health. Frequent contacts with him were of no avail but I just had to remain where I was and worsened my health.

The Coarse Black Snake:

I returned to Kumba after the Director had told me that he was going to take action later. I was sitting in the parlour till eleven thirty p. m. Then I left for my bed. I lied down gradually on my back but putting my head gently on my pillow. In a second, I heard a hissing noise. I raised up my head and it continued. I got up quickly. It must be a snake I said. I got my lamp and on looking, I saw a hideous snake, black and with a coarse body lying under the pillow but with its head pointing upwards ready to bite. I got a stick and a lance. I said I must be Sir Lanceleot. [42]. As soon as I moved where it was it glided under the bed and disappeared. I left the bed room alone and sleep in my parlour with a panting heart.

The transfer:

It is quite clear that my investigations were now having firm grounds when the Doctor recommended that I should change environments. People amused themselves by making expensive jokes about myself and the transfer. Each time I was going to work the voices of people around, not voices of spirits again echoed [43]: "Transfer me and my Sanger radio to Sasse school". When I was leaving the office for the house same echoe again of voices would repeat: "Transfer me and Molulu Sanger to my Sasse house." There was nothing so vital to me again other than my transfer as I was getting fed up with nuisances everywhere in the Church, along the streets, in the market and in my bed while asleep. Even in my house there were still people who found it a necessity to disturb me. All the nick-names in Kumba were given to me but the only thing that moved me to pity was my ill-health. All what I know was that some of the people have not learned to live in their own ways.

The transfer was changed to the Balondos Transfer. Although I was often in grief with pain and with what I had not yet known about my illness, I was often amused at the remarks of the people [44]. Although I was alone, yet other people declared themselves Balondos and so I was backed up by the "Balondos on foot and some Balondos in cars." It became known to everyone that "the Balondos transfers" are always a problem to them because despite the Doctor's recommendation for an immediate transfer, my TRANSFER WAS delayed for six months.

I could not understand what people expected me to do because no one ever met me and told me something about what they wanted of me. I was always thinking for myself and was trying by all means to do what I could; yet those who disagreed never came out plainly but often in disguise and their feelings, were all burried in them. Only empty talking merely to confuse a seculated person who was trying to leave to a standard suitable to himself so as not to involve himself into social problems which were above his little capacity. It was nothing but a social insanity because I was often scorned by many who said they were transferring me to my house or office, if I was facing any of these directions either a car, a motor cycle, a pedestrian and all what would pass me on the way and whosoever was riding said he was transfering me to where I was going. These should really have no place here but because the people concerned have to make amendments, I find it necessary for it to be stated here.

In fact, the year 1968 was the year that all things went bad with me. Whenever I met people for some private consultation people thought that I was negotiating to get money from them or that I was reporting them. If I were going to Buea, Great Kumba thought that I was going to report them because my examples and reports to the police about what was happening to me had disciplined the town. I was "singled out" in the town and everything about me was known by everyone, small or big [45], but I was not worried for any good thing done has a reward although sometime it may not be material.

At last I struggled and my transfer came through and I left the place peacefully and set my back to what had happened to me [46].

Medical Examination:

I wanted to know what had become of me after such long torture. It was discovered that all the disturbances had broken down my nervous system. Other effects of this were internal and abdominal pains, frequent occurences of images in my eyes at the back of my mind, some movement inside my skull. These are still very common now.

The Native Doctor:

Before I had my medical examination I also consulted the native Doctor [46] who gave me some treatment and some medicine to use in future. This too was very helpful and he hopes to attend to me any time I go up to him.

Reaction of the Public:

The action of the public has taught me a great deal. It has proved to me that something was really done by a set of people for their own interest. The same signs which occurred in many other places exist wherever I go and this tells me how much they have known from me by their supernatural ways and that if I have learnt something from them it might have been of some help to me. They have often been suggesting to draw a parallel from me.

Conceptions:

Many people have their own conceptions so that if the conceptions of everyone are presented they will give a very vague idea of me because they said they were giving me a national character [47]. The drama has been a national one in as much as grunts, murmurs, similar echoes, catch words or what they term their "I was" scorns, are principal features of their national character.

Proof that it was a planned act to dissociate me from my friends and the community:

At Kumba, actions and behaviour of the people around showed that they knew what was wrong with me but none of them came round to tell me. When I was stricken by the plague, I saw someone along the road who said, "you are now a big man." Therefore he knew what had happened but was not willing to tell me anything.

2. Words, expressions in English and my vernacular relating to my actions in the house and in the office are a sure proof.

3. Before this, the name Lonka had reigned in the vicinity. This only helped to add more fire to the situation. If there had been closer contact between the sufferer and the amused public, the pressure of torture on him would have been lessened. God knows our most secret thoughts but what I thought was conveyed to the public [48], but not such conveyance of their own thoughts was led to me. ThereforeI was merely used as a wall or an object against which each individual casts or reflects his thoughts.

4. Attitude of the public at church services or at private time in church and when boarding a vehicle to a destination give a clue to this.

5. Although the scene of happening was predominant in the set-up disturbances; yet everywhere I went: - hospital, Chemist shop, etc. I received the same tortures which were displeasing to the affected nervous system. Noise was not pleasing to my ear and to my mind. I did not make it so but illness. There was a type of noise that was made specially when I was around. I does not mean that ordinary noise which had no bearing with me offended me. Why did special noise offend me? Because most people or all those who use that type of telepathy [49] refused to tell a sick man exactly what was the meaning of what had happened to him, particularly as it all referred to me. It was an attempt to make me a fool and to obey like a parrot.

6. All such meaningless sounds or expressions as "Phom Fool", "Yu Bibil", "Sulelele", you "phom fool", were common everywhere I went.

7. My movements through the East and West have shown me that those expressions which are not at all mentioned here were all the same. It happened that whenever I came to a town, I would be led by some voices to a long distance out of the town before they eventually died out.

8. I thought of many things and in a second, I heard people commenting on my thoughts [50] some distance far off. These are just a few points in which I expressed my opinion about what man has done. This is the falacy of man. It does not pay anybody a cubic of an inch to suffer another soul without a good reason. Even if there is a good reason the person should know so that he can bear the sufferings patiently but man will not like to work where he will not harvest.

We can be doing good to ourselves if fault-finders are given this type of torture but not innoncent individuals. But we should know that another man's meat is another Man's poison. People are not of the same tastes [51].

It sounds unbelievable for something to spread out like wild fire among all men from the list to the greatest about a few persons. When some people are suffering others take so much pleasure and go gay to worsen the situation. It means that in such a society no progress exists but retrogression. A backward society must be carefully handled by its leaders and bad practices should be stamped out.

In concluding, I will live to say that man proposes but God disposes. Seeing the much long suffering I have undergone and still more fresh in me, I am not afraid if I do what I will especially as people of highlight merely feminine set will not just tell me my faults. The whole phase of this story is in connection with witchraft in our society, and the writer has been deliberating on a small narrative which he believes is connected with Black art that may have a fatal influence on man. He dwells all the time with particular reference to himself as an eye witness to some affliction that occured to him. "Do what you think, all things love me" [52].

Patient was transfered to Bamenda; but there was no difference. More torture was experienced - hence the Doctor recommended for another transfer. - See second part of story.

PART II: DISEASES AND WITCHCRAFT IN OUR SOCIETY - A PLAY

This is a typical insight of the happenings in a society. It is not uncommon that a thing started by a few or a small group of persons in a remote quarter spreads all over like a contagious disease. Although this may seem secret at the start or buried in our thoughts; yet the good or evil secret circulates round through various outlets. Any point that may be raised for or against this mood of affairs is conflicting because it scorches people's minds as to the source of revelation of the secret. The question arises now. How do we live in this World? Are we governed by spirits? In this case, one may be posed for some time to believe that some sort of spiritualism or witchcraft practice and by this agency information is carried like lightning from pole to pole.

Some psychological punishment originated through either the generous or selfish aims of some people may be administered on a group or on an individual through this means. This will also reveal to us that our earth is a paradise of rebellion, rebellions in thoughts, rebellions in our work and in fact every action of man may be rebellious in one thing or the other. No body will deny the fact that our troubles on earth usually start in this form. This story which is turned into a play is also going to tell us how people live. You will learn about good people, bad people, good spirits and evil spirits. There is nothing doubting from my own point of reasoning that we are not completely separated from our ancestors who died many thousands of years ago.

This play is going to tell us how some innocent people bear calumnies [53] intended by the others to mar them from all aspects of life or to probject [54] them as stars or notorious outlaws. Anyway, we do not want fools in our country and so people should not be made to behave like fools. Some scenes in this play may be very lively as there is humour throughout but in others there is very little or no talking at all and this imposes dullness on the scenes. But I can assure you that when you try to understand the train of the play and once you got this idea, the silent scenes are just as lively as the others. However, whatever your judgement may be at the end, I do hope you will appreciate this and bring up your criticism in writing, so that it may help the writer to make adjustments where necessary.

As I mentioned earlier, it has finally resulted, from various pressures from the populus that the intended sufferer automatically falls seriously ill and has to move from Doctor to Doctor, consult Native Doctors and the intensity of this urges him to go round the length and breath [54] of his country.

THE MINISTRY OF FRAUD

A PLAY - THE COURT

The Prime Minister's visit to Kumba early in 1968 is of vital importance to the population. It was his maiden visit to this Division. The visit was so pleasing to everyone although I was not opportuned to see him.

The Prime Minister's appointment was a coincidence to my knowledge about Solomon the Wise of the old testament [55]. I was an interested reader of the Plain Truth [56] and much was written about King Solomon the Wise, his reign, foresight and wise judgement. At the time of the visit, the atmosphere was cloudy, rumours and conversations in our neighbourhood and around were centred round my deep interest in the Plain Truth.

What did this portray to me? I deduced that some people believed that my readings about King Solomon led to the appointment of our prime Minister whose name is also SOLOMON. "Enobii you done get your Prime Minister from your war alone from your Plain Truth readings. You see how weh God Edeh work for ground." This was so surprising to me for people to translate my readings into different dreams. How did these people know that I was reading the Plain Truth? After all, I never used to go to the public and announced that I was a reader fof the Plain Truth. How does this come about? Was I being espionaged in some spiritual way or how can that be possible? There is no smoke without fire. Therefore, these people are right in reasoning that way.

Insincerity, foul language and misuse of other names is pure fraud. Punning on a person's name carelessly is usually dangerous. This spreads like wild fire and its sources are its leaders. It is often difficult to find out such nuisances. The fraud spreads through the whole country within a short space of time and causes disaster to many if it is not checked.

The Head of this Ministry is usually hidden because its purpose is to destroy a pleasant society. His information reflects onto the people like the Sun's rays but steps can be taken to get rid of such a person.

If one can cast his/her thoughts on today's rummours and gossips he will gather a great deal. This not only blackens a society but also the souls of people. It is so fascinating when one enters a market, it is just the same when one loiters around a school, or elsewhere; little ones, men gossip; gossip, rummours, slander poisons the air around.

The talk poisons one's mind especially the minds of the imature, who are not strong to carry the world on their shoulders.

Characterisation

Some of the characters in this play are alive, others are dead but happen to come back to life to comfort a patient. But one can always look or imagine a good spirit to be like an angel, a bad one to be like Satan or Lucifer. However, since these characters are living we are going to make them behave as they do when alive and the others who are really spirits and probably have never been met in life should behave like the angels and Satan.

As the characters are many, a brief account of the most important ones is here underneath sketched out. It is difficult to say something about each character and as this is mentioned in the play there is no place here for repitition.

The names that appear here, I say again, are those who have done very much in the play or have met the heroe from time to time giving him their views about the matter at stake. The heroe here is the man around which the story is centred. They are really two persons [57] shouldering the pains or sweetness of the story and other characters arise as a result of relationship in social circles of different aspects of life. The heroeine too as you may guess is in the same soup with the heroe although the latter champions the play.

The two big figures are in love and their dear and respectful relationship is translated into envy, jealousy and hatred and they are tantalised, jeered at wherever they happen to go. They are criticised, scorned and the use of foul language and pedantic [58] expressions, lulled them to stage clowns and sometime they look foolish among the other citizens because they, the citizens alone know what they have done. The story of this spreads out through the whole country and everywhere children and men know all about the persons most affected in the play.

The situation is very bitter to the men of good will and to the persons to whom this is intended and from the start it looks as though the story will be a tragedy but the constancy of the heroe and heroine mysteriously transforms the play into a comedy [59] and this brings joy to many. In fact nobody reads the thoughts of two friendly persons [60]. Through irritations of others, they may become bitter against each other and as soon as they are together each one laughs the sorrow and torments to scorn.

However, what seemed to be taken away from these persons is seen to be yielding fruits and everyone now judged his conscience and soon discovers that he/she was merely obeying like a parrot and did not know what he/she was doing.

In the end the two persons are rewarded for their bravery and constancy and while the "he" goes ahead in search of the golden fleece [61] the "she" has to stay for some time before going to rejoin her companion.

Characters:

Tipuan (the Demon):	A man with a forceful voice and with a good knowledge of the society. Alert and full of fun and mixes up with people of different walks of life. Knows the alphabet. Not alive.
Aja (the Demon):	A man of six feet fall, light in complexion and full of athletic stunts. Has a reflective memory and fun of swimming with the snake. Speaks broken English. Not alive.
Mr. Andela:	Likes to be in suit, speaks with ease but not too freely. Has gentle looks and smiles freely when amused.
Dr. Lantum:	Tall, lean, dark in complexion, smart in movement and takes long strides. Speaks good English and Fluently. Can use the professional language very well. Strict at his work and views a sick case critically and sympathetically.
Mrs. Lantum:	Well read and can speak both English and French; co-operative and encourages Co-operation. She is fluent.
Dr. Schwarz:	Of European accent [62]. Tall and gentle and takes interest in all his patients and also hardworking.
Dr. Muna:	Tall and lean and dark in complexion. Kind and takes interest in all his patients and also hardworking.
Fr. Sullivan:	Of European accent. Full of the knowledge of life and of the world. A religious man. Well educated and full of good counsel, sympathetic and always ready to listen to everyone. He is social.
Betty:	Speaks good English and fluently. Easily excited or moved to action. Can sing very well and also very flexible. Likes friends, gentle.
Kits [63]:	Kind, religious, trustworthy. Has a serious but gentle countenance and mixes with any type of persons. A very good Athlete.
Rose:	She is tall, lean, light in complexion, and feels very conservative with her "friend". Has motherly looks and is very gentle. Has a gentle and dignified speech and speaks with a low voice. The heroine of the play. Very patient. A good Athlete and also religious [64].

Fontem:	Smart movement, tall, lean and can display with her tongue. Business minded and argumentative. She can bully. Can sing well; also floats.
Patient Tanka: [65]	The central figure of the play (heroe). Easily moved to pity. Business minded. Religious; can become argumentative if not satisfied or wronged in anything. This is a weak point in his character, as people take this as an undue advantage to pull him out of the tone of gentleness. Has a very strong character but this is envied by many. Looks with equality, on everyone, is very conservative. His girl is his Queen hence he must be strict and patient.
Bridget Awasum:	Lean tall, quite, always ready to give a helping hand. (But as far as this story is concerned she appears in a different form and consequently her whole character sketch can not be revealed here.) Interested in people.
Simon:	Not Educated but is full of valour especially at Kumba where patient is visited in spiritual form by his three brothers as mentioned in the play. He takes active part in the snake and kneel fight [66] in the town in an onslaught. As an ordinary man he shows the deepest and brotherly love to patient and visits him in his sick bed in many occasions while at home, patient is sheltered by him and is always willing and always at his disposal. Simple and gentle and talks little. Has a deep interest in his associates.
Joe:	Kind, sympathetic and always ready to give a helping hand. A Good disciplinarian, business minded and feels at home with his friends.
E.O. Mrs. Nkembe:	Expresses motherly feelings, sympathetic and always ready to help where necessary but as a civil servant is very strict with proceedure. Patient and handworking [67].
E. O. Elonge:	Reading his fifties but looks energetic and of medium height. Takes interest in growing his hair tall. Always serious at any little thing and easily offended. If he hates you, then he has hated you all the time. Talkertive and shuns any long discussions which he usually terms arguements. A good musician and often praises his children.

Sister Aquinas:	Full of motherly grace and wisdom, interested in patients and children and gives good and religious counsel. Patient never saw her, but she spoke loudly to him and introduced herself to be Mother Aquinas. As far as this is concerned and since a spirit can take any form and speech, nobody knows except God and "those" concerned whether it were these people who were really speaking to the abandoned patient.
Father John:	Religious and full of common sense. Convincible and a great orator. Of European accent and may be reading his fifties but full of energy.
Helen:	Young looking and reserved, interested in friends and has very little to say when patient narrates his troubles to her personally. But at the time of incidence appears in a different form advising patient in a spiritual form and patient feels movement on his body. Sympathetic and considerate to everyone.
President:	Patient sees only his shadow and hears his speech. Stately in appearance and wears a white gown and a white cap. Friendly (by his visit and hand shake in his form).
Prime Minister:	In this form, patient hears a voice full of command. As a man he is tall, full of stately virtues.
Dr. Endelay [68]:	Appear to patient in spiritual form. Full of European fashion, tall, gentle looks and very experienced in the political world. From his actions in that form his kindness and respectfullness is portrayed.
Conny Van Zanten [69]:	Of European accent. Friendly and fun of sight seeing. Very gentle and blooming with beauty. Full of Courtesy. Always ready to help. But these qualities are actually shown in a mysterious form to patient in his sick bed.
Patient's Father AND Mother:	Extreme fatherly and motherly love, shares in patient's problems throughout.
Senior Education Officer, Mr. Ngwa:	Can not easily be convinced except by higher authorities, looks somewhat stern and hardly laughs except with his equals. Follows up matters very officially and restrains from using his initiative except when sanctioned from reliable quarters.
Bridget:	Plain and simple, very small girl of 12 years old, obedient and witty. Smart and can read a little.

Florence: Speaks pidgin and her tongue fluently. Sympathetic. A typical Country girl and respectful.

Mr. Kegham (Native Doctor): A man of medium height and probably in his fifties. Speaks neither English nor Pidgin. Full of enviromental sociology and never laughs. Speaks his tongue fluently which is translated by an interpreter. Has many wives and grandsons, daughters in his compound. His compound always full of patients.

Mr. Lucas (Native Doctor): Stout, quiet and with a large stomach. Speaks broken good English and when gambling he invokes spirits, chews some medicine in his mouth, strikes the table from time to time and whispers to his spirits. Before he starts gambling he looks at the patient's palm and from this he predicts many things. His is kind to his patients.

Mr. Mpah (Native Doctor): Stout, smart and a man of medium height. Views a sick case with great concern and sympathy. He is quite conversant to different type of illnesses and follows up his diagnosis critically and in rounds. Always ready to look into a case and "interested in people."

Ndikaka [70]: Related to Kegham. A medical worker and speaks good English, takes deep interest in people at first sight. A man of middle age, short and looks brave.

Sister Praidaig: Lives where the incidence occurs but appears to patient in an invisible form. Patient is made to believe this when an invisible person introduced her to him. Gives godly Counsel and full of European accent. In the fight which issued she exhibits bravery and constancy, seems daring and business minded [71].

Sister Antonia: Appearing in the same form as above but is well experienced. Encouraging and observant.

A POEM ON LOVE

O lady O lady
Thy silence tears away my heart like a hawk buchers a chicken.
Let the announcement of thy love flow like the waters of a fall.
Hasten, Hasten, O dearest one to visit they love in bed [72].

Knowest thou that the path of glory, leads but to the grave?
Knowest too that the path of love is full of rocks and thorns?
Thou seem not to see the rolling hours nor the bright sun from
East to West.

It's not a car that lags you behind.
It's not shyness that prolongs the announcement.
For thou art full of logic and maturity.
But the carefree friends and slander keep you away.

Love knows no pleasure in miniature.
It knocks with force at it's door.
Solve therefore thy problems with a simple mind.
For the luxury of love may be after marriage.

O, thou art not a munament
Unfold therefore the passion of thy love.
Speak in words and melody.
You are not a pig nor a goat that grunts and bleats.

Humming, the bee loves the flower,
The booming heavens signify thunder;
Interpret therefore thy love as human.
Ah! I cannot longer wait.

It's burning desire grows strong in me.
Why thinkest thou, you are slow to strike,
Echoe therefore my dreams in words and visits,
To shun the foolery of slander away.

While my socks slip down from my legs, and my sleeves left unbottoned [73].
Is not this because love is slow to spring?
Time gallops with the girl who sits and smiles like a munament [74];
And amples [74a] with the alert girl who seizes the opportunity at a stroke.

Carve [75] and sing thy verses in trees and stones.
Imprint them on thy face to glitter;
Let thy love not be so full of weariness and confussion.
If thou can't do this, if thou hast none of the above
qualities then thou has no love.
Thou must rest in peace [76].

Thou has no love, thou must learn to love
Let the air now come out of the bladder [77].
So that thy heart smiles at every one.
And thy love to keep in peace
And the war that should last lone may end.

Thy actions are passive and seem meaningless
Let them cheer up thy true spirits like spirit in wine.
Not in actions only nor in sound can you stand,
Because they will miscomprehend them
Therefore let them flow from the glory of they heart,
To heel thy wounded heart.

Why make thy love the hatred of the world?
Fight with a conscious mind to gain,

Pour not forth onto thy loved one thy wisdom in spirits,
For thou art not the wisest in the world
If thou love the world you live in work not therefore
with supernatural powers;
For this belittles you amoungst other men.

When stricken by shyness take him to the secret room.
Reveal thy thoughts to shame the world around.
Your mind goes dark every minute.
If thou cannot, thou art a murderer in such ways.
Thou should not pretend and do the wrong.
Miniature [78] love better fold thy arms and give up.

Oh! most modern love two years in bed [79]; thy love in anguish.
Modern days, modern fashion. Art thou the world's famous lover?
Therefore enlighten thy loved one, educate him.
Frowning, silence, disgust only wears away life from you.
Thou knowest much from the old and literate.
Why don't you shoot forth lika a young plant?
Growest then from fifty to thirty, or from thirty to fifty?
Yes, you want to carry five tons at one, instead of at five.
It's good to learn from the learned;
It's not good to know all what the learned knows,
This will make the world a dull place for the adolescence.

Oh Lord, I am embraced by thy rays and engulfed in thy arms,
Like an ant I adore you; in the midst of difficulties.
Thou commandest not only an ant but the giant too.
Who is then the greatest of men?
Thou commandest man not to death only, but to the greatest.
Therefore the nobles and plebians are thy servants.
What is man then; is not he just an empty breath?

Now, man thou art nothing but dust
Position and apparel maketh you not different,
The kitchen knave [80] and you are not same on earth;
But on the right hand of God thou art the same [81].
Bring not therefore chaos amoungst [81a] men of good will;
Segregation comes early in our society.
Men may be defined for sake of peace.
But in education and employment thy measures must not give way
To those by the way side.
Good speech, contact and corporation [82] will yield fruits,
For the physicians of growing nations are leaders and the law.

The seconds, months and years wear life from you,
Thou hast set thy men to arms and strike
Why standest therefore aside; the world will laugh at you.
The hearts of men have been enlightened by torture;
Open the springs of the mountain to cool them.

If thou cannot thou art a war monger.
Seest thou the reactions of thy men everywhere?
Seek therefore for means to satisfy them.
Let Tom be told of his mission and Dick of his agony.
Overshadow him not with nation's slander and super expirience,
Because this betrays you and your tacts amongst men.
If thou cant solve the problems of thy son,
Why put the sons of the plebians under the yolk of the nation?

These days are bitter days.
Our nation is young, although African imaturity of foresight
May lead us astray,
Scan thy tribes, the well read, with an experienced eye.
Cast therefore thy thoughts through the right angle.
Take time, acute angles are difficult and dangerous.
But they are the up springs, they like no torture.
Torture without a bearing is injustice
No mother, no father, offers a stone to a child that needs a fish.
No snake shares same hole with a "poukin pine" [83]
It's not threats nor slander to cheer up the child
That lags behind, but good counsel.

A goat fed in custody differs from the free one in forest.
If thou trust thy child offer him the education he wishes.
Suck not the blood from his veins before thy decision.
No girl marries at eight; Why therefore unfold life at a hundred
to a child of twenty?
Is not this a mental problem and isolation from life?
If thou art not a bully examine thy conscience in a lone monastry.

For how long do the booming heavens warn before thunder?
Within seconds and minutes comes the thunder.
Reason? Man is reasonable not a stone.
Warn a stone by breaking or rolling it away.
Warn thy son in words, as actions and signs may misinterpret you.
Dreams may bring suspicion and spoil thy child.
Therefore express thyself, speak to thy child in words.
Not in the way thou will train a bird in the zoo.
For this reveals self egoism and dislikeness of a different up-spring.

Oh Divine grace and lover of thy creature,
Infuse the liquid of peace into my scorched mind.
Brush the horizons of thy little intellect.
Inject the blood of life to purge the impurities that wind,
The deeps to install the poisons of the Devil. [84]

Protection of the Needy in Distress

1. O Capital, O capital emblem of Cameroon Occidental.
   Thy teeth point out like the shoot of a young Olive tree.
   From them we learn to grow in peace.
   But life seems to shake our minds and bones away from you.

2. Yet thou art the brightest star in the west.
   We do not know when the trumpet blows for end of time.
   But we hope to see the centuries ahead.
   We grow rich in Education in lifts and bounds [85].
   In chaos we shall be if we misinterpret the day and the future.

3. Lo! therefore extend thy arms to govern and engulf everyone.
   And pour forth thy icy fluid onto our heads.
   Neither creed, nor race be left asunder.
   For these thy gloomy days let the stars pray for us.

The Headquarters of this particular Fraud is centred around Kumba although it spreads to its neighbouring town Bamenda. Other places may be affected but these are the chief centres.

It began from the house of one Mr. B. N. Tanka. The Prime Minister giving commands in the evening at about 8 p.m. As the command was obeyed a series of other events occured beginning from the house to the church, and from the church to the market and back to the house. The same thing continued from the house again (to the house) to the office.

In fact, the whole day was marked by a series of events which continued until the next morning. It looked somewhat like a plague to the sufferer although not recognisable by those who met him. Even the District Doctor did not know this when he appeared to him for treatment.

The issue is presented to Dr. C. D. C. Hospital, who directed it to Acha Tugi hospital for treatment. The treatment lasted for two weeks and the patient is a little relieved but still being very conscious of his health contacted a native Doctor for more medicine and explanation. The story goes down again to Kumba and Tiko and at Kumba the patient is marred and tormented by the society. This leads to his recomendation for transfer to a place which appeared to have been aware of the situation [86]. The patient is impatient and gets nervous and finds everything as before whenever he goes. He takes a medical examination. He complaints to the District Doctor for a possible change of condition.

SCENE I

CRIME: INTIMADATION

Chief Justice: As the story goes, did you in any form not visible to the complainant appeare in his house at Kumba at 8 p.m. on the 20th March 1968?

Prime Minister: This is serious and strange. It needs a lot of thinking and investigation. It is difficult to say yes or no until we find it out by all possible means. Can you give me enough time to investigate this, my lord chief Justice?

Chief Justice: You should investigate this seriously because the law will not hesitate to measure drastic punishment to such acts of offences which are performed under the pretext of higher powers to inroot the discipline of good citizens and plant evil into the society.

Chief Justice: Can you read any Text from the law to support the statements just made above?

Barrister: In 1484, Pope Innocent VII passed "summis Desiderantees, the use of force to extract evil guilt on witchcraft in confession." In 1736 in America people were executed because of the use of high powers.

Chief Justice: Do you know anything concerning the above? And do you believe to have entered the complainant's body by any means between the hours of 12 and 1 and while moving in his body, you altered [87] these words: "I am Mr. Andela Speaking to you. When I speak do not speak, only listen. I am here with Dr. Lantum." Were you really in bis body or you played a trick to intimidate him. He complained of feeling much pains from your prickings and movement. Adding, the complainant says he recognized two shadowy figures by the side of his bed exactly your resemblance and that of Doctor Lantum.

Mr. Andela: Well, as I can very well remember, this child came to me looking pale and unconscious and I was not happy at his sight. He told me a similar story but I told him I knew nothing about it. I myself have heard rummours about this. I have known him to be reliable right from school and I had often met him during holidays when I was still in the University. Some of my friends know him to be somebody who hardly tells lies. As he persits [88] about what happens to him, I am sure he must have experienced something which was beyond his understanding as an ordinary man. And concluding, I hold fast with what the Prime Minister said earlier: that this is a matter to be investigated.

Chief Justice: What steps did you take further to find out what was wrong with him after he had left you?

Mr. Andela: As I said earlier his story was quite unatural to me and was very funny.

Chief Justice: Are you aware of this situation? That on a set day which I have just mentioned you performed some act of spiritual power to exhibit superiority of intellect and experience over this complainant. That in this form you communicated with him from any distance and that he heard your speech but could not see you. Sometime you spoke within his body and at other times you spoke from above. What was your object of such a hideous move by which you found it as a means to advise him, criticise him and talk to him angrily instead of sitting down with him and discussing these things over a bottle of beer? As I said earlier, this is a very serious crime and I am going to step into it and view with the highest regard of concern. I will not like such hideous deeds to be implanted into this young society.

Landa A: Your worship, this is something very funny and peculiar to me. In fact, I know this gentleman and many a time I do meet him. There can be no other way I can approach him than in this form, I am in front of you today. If this be a miracle it might have been wrought by some other person [89]. I cannot say anything more about this as my mind is too young, for the knowledge of the world it cannot bear.

Chief Justice: Is it a custom in the catholic Church as a whole or only in Kumba TOWN Church that people are criticised at prayer or being told what to do?

Priest: This is a funny question. Personally I have not withnessed such a thing.

Chief Justice: But this fellow in front of me tells me that he was disturbed by a series of voices at prayer in the church. For the whole time he was confused, misled and became unconscious at the end of the Service. Was that a type of punishment or teaching measured unto him?

Priest: Yes, I know him and he told me something of the sort but I could not understand the world. It may be someone wrought a spell on him. All I could tell him was that there was something wrong with his mind and I refered him to Doctor Lantum as he told me that the District Doctor did not know what was wrong with him.

Chief Justice: What were your findings when this child came to you?

Doctor: I saw no illness in him but I prescribed some medicine for him.

Chief Justice: Was that all you did for him?

Doctor: He came to me on several occasions for treatment. But on the second occasion, I told him that there was something wrong with his mind [90] but there was no specialist to whom I could recommend him. The other time he wanted me to give a medical Certificate to certify that he was ill but I did not do so.

Chief Justice: You as Doctor could not have refused to issue a sick medical Certificate to him after finding that he was ill. If there was no specialist in the country you should have given him that permit to seek for treatment elsewhere or asked his head of Dept. to help him get medical attention somewhere.

Doctor: Your worship, yes I should have done so but I received no letter or even a telephone message from the local Head of Dept.

Chief Justice: You as a Doctor have the right to recommend someone to abstain himself from duty or to go elsewhere for treatment as soon as you recognize that he is incapable of performing his duty because of ill-health. Have you anything to say?

Doctor: No, earlier I told you that I asked him verbally to seek the attention of any medical officer since there was no specialist in the country to do this.

Chief Justice: Is that the proceedure, and how was he to carry this out? On his own private expenses or on Government expense?

Doctor: Either means but as a civil servant the Government could help to treat him.

Chief Justice: How have you been receiving your treatment? Is it on your own expenses or Government?

Complainant: On personal expenses.

Chief Justice: This is someone who was helping you and offering his services to the Government and to his country. You saw him ill and he came up to you complaining. What steps did you take as a local head of Dept. to get him well?

Education Officer: I asked him to go to the Doctor but I refused to write a note or telephone to the Doctor.

Chief Justice: What did he tell you later?

Education Officer: He told me that the Doctor refused to give him excuse duty permit or to recommend him to any other Doctor.

Chief Justice: You representing the Government in your Dept. in this area is responsible for the welfare of anyone working under you, not so? That is one of your duties. On hearing this what measures did you take to let him seek the Doctor's attention?

Chief Justice: You were not exercising your duties as a local head of Dept. You are probably misusing the power which is given to you and it will appear that you know something concerning the illness of this fellow or otherwise you have a biassed mind about his own welfare. Meanwhile this matter is still under strict investigation and you may still be called up to say more when the findings are out.

SCENE II

Inside the patient's House someone who introduces herself to be Sister Aquinas is speaking on his head. He gets a mirror and a comb to find out what was making such distinct speech on his head but he sees nothing. However, the voice advises him to sit down and get some beer ready for his father and some members of his family who were coming round. He is soon interrupted by friend Mr. Tonna.

"THE FEAST"

Things Present: Two loaves of butter bread, dining table, one bottle of small guinness stout, one bottle of grenadin, a tin of margarine, a glass, cutlery.

Patient: Sitting at table in his house obeying spirits and feasting. During this period he is being advised by Mr. Andela:-

"Be very careful in this place. Do not be afraid. Eat gently and do not fear that any person will do anything wrong to you. I shall speak to your boss and she will do no harm to you." (Here someone hiding should be speaking or advising to represent the spirit). After feast is over, same spirit leads patient to office talking to him all the time. Advising, warning, etc.

"Move along the main road and let's see who will give you a lift, as many people say here that they know you. As I am speaking to you, try to move in rhythm with my speech. Pay attention to me. All your friends are here with me but as your eyes are not yet opened you cannot see us." A small tiny fly lands on his body and pierces into his body. It introduces itself to be Dr. Lantum. Mr. Tona comes in, also in human form.

Mr. Tona: What is actually wrong with you?

Patient: I heard some voices of invisible and mysterious persons in my body. Others were speaking above but I did not see those who were speaking. Yesterday too was my feast day. I had given some money to the priest to say some mass for me and my friends. As I was going to church, I was disturbed by some voices. Even when I was entering the church I was criticised and tormented mercilessly. Really the whole of yesterday, I was not at rest. In my house, in the church and in the office and wherever I went.

Mr. Tona: How were you tormented?

Patient: Some of the voices were heard in me and there was a painful and piercing movement through my veins. As this happened something was dropping from the inside walls of my body. In fact, something like blood. This weakens my nerves and my thinking system [91].

Mr. Tona: Did you see the priest?

Patient: Yes, I did so and he even came here and blessed this house. Please Mr. Tona I will no longer stand any more questioning from you. I am so tired.

Mr. Tona: Do not think so much but pray and try to see the Doctor tomorrow.

Patient: The Doctor says I am not sick. He gave me some tablets only. I can't help thinking. I have been induced to think so very unnecessarily by the incidence. Probably there is a poison in my blood.

Mr. Tona: Just be patient and do not be woried. (He gets out of his seat and walks towards the front door)

Patient: Also gets out of his seat and sees him off. "Good night and thank you very much."

SCENE III

Inside Patient's House: Heard the sound of a moving car. The car soon came to a stop. Something in an invisible form spoke on his head, about the arrival of the Reverend Sister: "I am here in a different form, I am coming in my human form to you soon."

Patient: Gets nervous and was anxiously waiting to see the said visitors. Meanwhile he has sent already for the beer as ordered by the spiritual form of Sister Aquinas. The beer is soon brought in but in vain did any body come in?

Sister Aquinas: I am the Principal in charge of all Catholic girls secondary Schools in West Cameroon. You should be very careful with yourself. Do you know one girl by name Rose in our Lady of Lourdes College, Monkon?

Patient: (Right from the onset patient has been asked never to speak but to listen).

Sister Aquinas: You should not feel that you are alone in the house. (In saying this two other Reverend Sisters came in namely Sister Antonia and Sister Praidaig, Principal of girls Training Centre, Fiango).

Sister Aquinas: I will like to stay with you and teach you English. Get a bottle of beer and drink.

Patient: (Calls out his brother for a bottle or beer and a glass.)

Sister Aquinas: Advises patient in that unknown form, "I am getting information about all what is happening in Kumba and I will tell you later".

Sister Antonia: Get your clock.

Patient: (Gets the clock and places it on the table.)

Sister Antonia: I will enter the clock and speak to you. Pay great attention and you will hear my speech when the clock is ticking.

Patient: (He listens and hears something funny. The ticking of clock was like a speech.)

Sister Praidaig: I am giving you information about what is happening in Kumba. Be very careful with yourself.

Patient: (Feels sleepy and the sister advises him to go to bed.)

Sister Praidaig: I am well armed and dangerous and anyone who ventures to come round for evil, I will be stern on him.

Sister Praidaig: (Speaking angrily to an agressor.) What do you want here Mr. Elonge? Are you not ashamed of yourself to fight a woman in this form? I will deal with you because I am very dangerous at this moment. (As she was speaking I only heard the buzzing of wings as though some insects were fighting.)

Sister Praidaig: I have sent the intruder out. He will not more come here.

Patient's Father) A spirit informing patient that his parents will
Patient's SISTERS) be flown to Kumba in an helicopter.
Mr. Lawson)

Spirit: An helicopter has been flown from Victoria to your home to collect your father and your sisters to Kumba to see you.

Patient: (He is quiet. Can't ask any questions to invisible beings, as he looked on, he soon saw four shadows sitting down and this action was done briskly.)

Spirit: Your sisters are at the camp, where that girl's parents are, and your father has been taken down to Victoria by Mr. Lawson. You have just seen your sisters here in a different form and you will not see them again. Your father went down to Victoria with some money in his bag. A very heavy sum of money about 264,000 francs. I am afraid if he takes plenty of drink the money will be carried off.

Father Sullivan: I am still on leave in U.K. but I have heard and seen that you are ill, that is why I have come to visit you. I am here with two friends from Britain. We shall have to go into you and after that will examine you to know what is wrong with you. We shall also take some snap shot while you are sitting in your sleeping gown.

The Menka Demons: (Namely: Demon Aja Adu, Demon Tipuah, Demon Tashi, Demon Tabu and Demon Aku: Displaying acrobatic stunts by the wall).

Father Sullivan: Get a bottle of beer and drink, we shall also drink in our own way and you will not know.

Patient:(Sitting in his night dress and notices some flash of light under the table. This flash of light pierces through the table and enlarges.)

Examination by Londoneers:

Father Sullivan: We are examining you to see if there is something in you. We have also taken the snap shot.

Patient: (in the parlour alone in the evening about 8 p.m. Five shadowy figures of Demons appear carrying stones on their heads. They are taking exercise. They should stand erect against the wall.
Sit down in crouching positions with the stones on their heads, stretching their hands upwards, sideways, down-wards and pulling their muscles out.)

Demons: (One Demon speaking). This is how we used to play in School in those old German days. (Indicates this by carrying heavy loads on their heads, sitting down, raising their bodies up gradually and stretching their hands sideways.)

Demon Aja: I died a few months after your birth. I saw you but my elder brother who is here (he introduces him, a tall, dark complexion, 6 feet person still in his thirties). We are showing you how we used to play at school in our German Days, (he dramatises) how we used to play football in School or in my Village. There was no Youth who could stand with me. (He handels a snake by the neck and dived into a swimming pool.)

Patient: (Looks quietly at the Scene.)

Aja: We are demons and our speed is like lighting.. If we leave you know we will be within second and two in U.K. and America respectively. We have travelled to many parts of the World. We heard that you are ill and we have been advised by people at home to visit you. To show you that we know you, we must tell you the names of all those you know here in Kumba. (Here any series of names can be read to the patient to the hearing of the audience.)

Demon Tipuan: (A man of medium height 5 feet, 6 ins, light in complexion, wears a coat without a tie. Has a sharp, distinct and forceful voice. Usually speaks loudly.)

Demon Aja: (Swimming in a swimming pool holding a large snake by the hand.) This is how I used to swim, to develop my muscles. You will be taught how to swim with the snake when you go home and your backbone will be straightened on a bamboo and you will grow taller.

Tipuan: We the Demons have been to the parents of that girl and they seem difficult people to disclose their minds to us. Mark you, I have seen this girl in two occasions. In the first occasion I asked her of you and she said she knows you. I left her a message for you. In the second occasion, I appear to her in a School dormitory. You will be taught how to invoke when you go to your new Station. Someone in that School invoked me and the girl I appeared to her in a dream was a very close friend to you. Do not be doubtful because it is more easy for women to deal with Spirits than men.

Demons: (Coming forward altogether with a file. Opened and showed me all written about me by my boss. "Look at your file". (One of the demons speaking. Patient looks on the file and sees clearly his name written on it.)

Demons: (Reading my thoughts.)

Patient: (Recognises two and falls into deep thoughts.)

Demon: (Recalls patient back to his past deeds when alive. He strikes at once about five sticks of matches, this representing a gun shot to a visitor he folds his arms, looks at patient.) You are thinking about the voices you heard yesterday in this house and about the happening now in your house.

Demon Aku:(Of heavy voice, stout and light in complexion with a hairy body, wears a hat.) You are thinking about my name and that of Clement Tabu.

Patient:(Is dead silent and almost frozen in his chair as they say exactly what he thinks [92]).

Tipuan: (Warning) Leave this room. People are coming here for a meeting.

Patient:(Insists and sits down as he is tired to be hearing voices from spirits. He feels movement under his feet.)

Tipuan:(Speaking under patient feet but inside the floor.) I say again (shouting angrily) leave this room and go to your bedroom.

Patient: (Is left alone perplexed. He goes to his bedroom immediately.)

Demon Elias: (Tipuan's friend and former teacher to patient. Take time in this place, recalls himself to patient and told him all about him when he was at School.)

Demon Tabu and Aku: (They read my thoughts. Said out what I thought. Give some example e.g.) "you are thinking that we are dead men."

Demons altogether: We know all about you here in Kumba and about your examinations.

SCENE IV

Patient:(Sitting in the Parlour - he is soon induced to laugh at the sight of a figure which appears quite distinct in front of him. It walks towards him and vanishes. The figure of Rose.)

Spirit: (A spirit speaking in Patient)
That is the figure of a girl you know. She will be teaching at R.C.M. Buea Road, during the holiday.

Patient:(Is left alone and is frightened at night by three Ghosts.)

1st Ghost: (By recognition is Christine Fontem. This Ghost is slender and tall and appears to patient almost naked and a type of repugnant odour [93] is produced by the Ghost. It appears that the Ghost rubbed some sticky ointment on its body. The ghost climbed on the radio and walked speedily across the head bed. The patient's hair stands on end as he is frightened.)

2nd Ghost:(Another Ghost came in and bounced three times on the stomach of patient. It is very light in weight like the weight of a pumped bladder. By recognition, this was the Ghost of Betty.)

3rd Ghost: (The third Ghost was completely in the skin of a snake, a very nasty appearance. It lied down by the side of the patient. Beats its legs on the bed, gave a loud cry and fell under the bed. This was the ghost of Rose.)

Patient: (Is frightened the whole night and did not sleep at all. The next morning the radio went bad. Probably is damaged by the Ghost.)

Father Sullivan: (Advises; not in his human form but in his spritual form). Get your radio to the town for repairs and also get some money and go to Mr. Andela, the Secretary to the Prime Minister and tell him what has happened to you.

Patient: (Gets money and went to Buea. Goes to the inquiry where he fills a form to see Mr. Andela. Form is taken up.)

Patient: (Waiting for a call. He is called up. He goes in and Mr. Ake goes out.)

Patient: Good morning, Sir.

Mr. Andela: Good morning. Sit down. What do you want?

Patient: I saw something like a vision. I heard many persons in my body and moving in my veins causing much pains and others were speaking above but I saw nothing. I was interupted for the first part of the evening, between the hours of 12 and 1 o'clock, and also the following morning right from my house to the church and to the Office. In fact, the whole day was marked by much talking from spirits. I am still being disturbed by the talking within but not without now. This appears to me like a dream and one of the spirits has asked me to come to you for explaination.

Mr. Andela: I don't know anything about it, Mr. Tanka.

Patient: (Goes out with an unhappy and perplexed mind. He goes back to Kumba.)

SCENE V

Patient: (Gets home tired and sleeps early. In the night a lot of disturbances was made in the Gernadarms camp. All talking is relating to the happenings of his vision. Some say this, others say that, all types of very vague and disheartening language was very common and was merely to make the patient unhappy. The patient glances through the bed curtain and suddenly sees a white board on which were written the inscriptions:)

"Queen Elisabeth II." (After this, the figure of Queen Elizabeth appeared in transparent apparel. So majestical and distinct like coloured picture, it was. Myriads of shadowy figures were seen too.)

Someone: (Not probably a spirit, but a living person hiding in a house in the distant.)
"Mua qua-qua forty, Mua qua-qua forty," [94] said someone in the distance.

Patient: (Guessed the voices and seemed to know the persons around speaking. Then he said to himself): there must be something brewing around.

An Officer: (Most probably, who is believed to be questioning some girls and some women. The voice is heavy but not so distinct because of the distance.) What are you doing here at this time of the night? What type of noise are you making and what is the meaning of that? (This is what the patient thought the officer was saying to the girls and women.)

Patient: (Lying in bed during the day. Tension of Pains great and finds it difficult to sleep.)

Girl: (The sound of an angelic float [95] from a girl gives sweet music to patient. After floating the girl changes to singing (angelic). The singing wakes up the patient from sleep with a type of laughter. He looks up the ceiling where the music was coming but saw nothing. In addition he sees many other shadowy figures.)

Devils: (Reappear again. Whisper in patient's ears, speak loud. This appears to the patient as though the spirits were really shouting. Acrobatic stunts.)

Demon Tipuan: (Planting his feet into the earth, disappears and comes out from another corner. He is watched by his Demoness, an American girl.)

SCENE VI

Some noise made by people in the vicinity. The use of foul language and meaningless expressions such as Mua qua-qua forty.
"Your grave is behind your house. Mua-qua forty, there should be a symbol of a grave behind the house." This noise lasts only for about 3 minutes and is soon broken by a theatre of shadowy figures ranging from the least to the greatest man in the country. After this, steps in Demon Tipuan, singing and shouting. He danced from corner to corner, stands erect, plants his legs into the ground, disappears and comes out at the other end.

Display of Life History: Tipuan shows life history of patient right from infancy to the present moment. Here there should be a display of a baby, the time of crawling right up to school age and adulthood. The spirit Tipuan calls out all the names of patient's friends which he heard with great dismay.

The Resurrection: No body died and no body rose from the death. But it was likened to the resurrection in the bible. This goes to tell you the peoples opinion about the patient. Did they want him to recover, did they want him to die?

Someone: Boh, Is he not dead yet?
(Betty comes forward, beckons at patient and speaks in patient's native tongue but this speech was not clear to patient's ears. She looks with a pretentions love Scorn).

Dick: That man, can he ever die?

Someone: (There is a fine grave already dug behind his house, you can see it. Someone cleverly covered it up with grass. This is a true statement. There was really a small pit which someone has made but there was grass on it.)

Dick: He is dead because he is sick [96] and because his girl is away from him. Now when he shall be well it will be as he ressurected and this resurrection will be marked when he is with his girl.

Someone: We are really suffering this man. Imagine he cannot see us and we are really filling his mind with our thoughts [97] which I am sure are negative to him.

President Adhidjo: (The president steps forward in his white gown and offers sixteen thousand francs to someone in the crowd. At this offer noise came from the concentration camp:) That is money for your over Sasse Order [98]. (This speech is so touching to patient. He has finished with his order. But this gives a clue to patient of a possible plan that was organised to stupify him, His head is heavy with pains.)

In the Parlour: An Indian file of dancing men and women stepped before patient from back door showing him different presents which reflected his mind back to his past deeds, e.g. showing of pictures, letters, money etc. Crowd danced and sings in pidgin and goes out at the front door.

2nd Crowd: (Three persons step in like patient's brothers also singing in pidgin:) Na wee, na wee, We small, we small; for fight, We deh na witch na witch, we deh.
Anything, anything we go try. [99]
(Speech of song is so appaling to patient but he observes in perfect tranquility. Figures were distinct but not real persons.)

One of the Brothers: We are from home. We have heard that you are sick and that the people here seem not to like you. That is why we have come to see you.

3rd. Crowd: (Patient is sitting in the parlour and he sights another crowd. Two lawyers step in their official apparel, reading Voluminous books in silence. A third person is a former school mistress to patient while the former are School mates. The procession lasts for a few minutes and the images vanish.)

President: (Comes out of my bedroom in a light blue gown and a small white cap. He raises up his hand to shake with patient.)

Tipuan: (Sprang up from one corner like demonian guard and said:) I am a Demon. (He told a short story to the President in his life as a president.) I have been coming to your residence. Sometime ago you wanted to board a plane from Douala to some destination, but I got there and warned you not to go because there would be an accident on the road. Do you forget me and the time I admonished you not to go where you wanted to go?

President: I have not forgotten you.

Tipuan: As you are the head of State, can you allow me to come back to life?

President: I am also guarded by demons and never in the history of revelation has someone dead come back to life. (He waves his hand in the air indicating refusal to Tipuan's question; smiling at the same time. Facing the spirits and remarking about my house he said.) In many occasions I have been coming here for protection and I have found the house a suitable quiet place. (At this, the Ghosts vanish.)

Girl (Helen): (Advising patient to be careful with himself. This advise prolonged and patient was tired and became angry and the spirit girl disappears.)

The Demons Examination

Tipuan and his gang (seven spirits) come forward and threw certain things on patient's body. At this they said they were finding out what was wrong with him as they have heard much talk about him. Shaking of blood in veins and the effect of medicine forces blood to shake.

The Doctors Examination

It sounds foolish but patient hears movement and speeches in his body and three Doctors introduced themselves to him. They said they were examining him. (These are not visible but speech is heard.)

Identity in Voices: (Two girls known to the patient speaking from the distance. This may be imitation by some people but some spirit tells patient that they were the girls. A heavy, gentle soft but dignified voice probably indentifies one of the girls and the other distinct, but full of love must be the voice of the other.)

Motor Car glides along the Road: (A spirit informs patient of the owner of the car and that the girls were in the car.)

Patient: (He really heard the sound of voices and that of a car which came to a stop. Some people murmuring. He leaves the door ajar and was waiting to receive the visitors, but in vain; they failed to come.)

Patient: (Gets tired of waiting and goes to bed. He hears the footsteps of someone who moves fastly past the back door to the hedge near the kitchen and there he heard a sound as though something was thrown there. In the night, patient sees someone dressed like a Jew. Then he sees Tipuan by the window. He speaks through patient's ears telling him what was happening. The Jew is Saint Jude, [100] patient's Patron Saint for difficulties.)

St. Jude: I have been hearing your prayers. You should continue to pray. When I was young, I spent all my time praying and I was sociable wherever I went. We have politicians too in our own world, different countries which also carry on their own administration. In our country persons can only see God through application and after doing their penances. God is kind and excuses those who died pegans.

Tipuan: I have already crossed so many gates and I will soon see God though I died a pagan.

St. Jude: I have been in this world and still I like to come out and enjoy myself. I am out for justice and will not like to be suffered nor want someone to be suffered innocently. My main object had been justice when I was alive and right up till now as a saint I am strongly against those who are unjust. I am leaving you (he said as he walked up to my bed, and off he disappears).

The Embalment:(In the morning, patient goes out of the house and stands in front of the back door. He hears from a voice such words like) "Opaque", "Telepathy",(and)" Embalment".(Here someone hidden in the distance should say out these words to represent the spirit. If there is a loft [101] the voice should come from above so as to appear as though the spirit is speaking from the patient's head. The patient should really be sitting down and hearing commands from the spirits. The same person in the distant or in the loft should be announcing to the patient.)

1st. Spirit: I am Hon. Lafon. I have heard that you are ill and I have come to visit you. (The speaker should introduce his speech in pidgin and then change to good English.) Compe, how you be now? (Then start at once by saying that) I am Hon. Lafon etc . (As on first line above.)

2nd Spirit: (Should be high spirited and dignified and of English accent.) I am Hon. Jua. I have come to see you because I heard that you are ill. (Hon. Jua in the form of a fly finds difficulty in getting into patient's body and goes back.) I must be guilty of some crime. (He goes back to get some medicine and on return he enters patient's body.)

Spirit: Your mother will get through you from your left handside, and your father also will go through you from your right handside.

Shey: I am from Yoaunde. I have heard of your illness and have come yonder to pay a visit to you.(After saying this he goes through patient's body.)

Spirit: About fifty-two persons have gone through you. You are very brave and in short the bravest of those who have been embalmed with you.

Mother: This is nothing but murder, only two persons went through me when I was being embalmed. Your veins have been opened and weakened and this will trouble you a great deal (she speaks some grammar and vernacula still within me.)

Father: Only four persons went through me when I was being embalmed. Your own embalment is above everyone. (Speaks some grammar and vernacula.)

Spirit: There is a witchcraft called Nyamzjah; when a person transforms himself into it he can understand any language. That is why different people who went through you were able to read your thoughts and some even spoke your tongue and your parents spoke some good English.

Principal: (Saint Joseph's College Sasse, a tall slender European of English accent, appears in white shirt and white pair of shorts. He is in company with patient's relative, of medium height and size.)

Principal Speaking:(Showing eight hard oblong papers.)These are the certificates in question. They will be given to Betty on this evening. She and Rose will bring the Certificates to you in your house.
Some people have been getting information from letters in your box or elsewhere in your house by means of the snake. All books which you loaned out to persons, those that were stolen, will be brought to you by these girls.

Patient: (Feeling pains in his chest, something actually piercing through his vertebral organs. Glidding with great difficulty and accute pains like a long worm. Patient should be drinking and trying to stop the pains by pressing his chest on his knees.)

Spirit Speaking to Patient: That is the spirit of Lonka A, coming to you. Her spirit is trying your ability to bear the burden. It will be coming to stay with you for some time. This means you are being put to a test. This will last for short time.

Patient: (The spirit of patient's father came to him.)

Spirit: You are now with the spirit of your father and it will be with you for the whole of today.

Patient:(His right eye winks and the spirit of Lonka A and father went out together and patient notices a white cloud going out through his right eye into heaven.)

Spirit: The spirit of Lonka also stays with Mr. Maimo. It appears you are calm and can bear the burden for a much longer period than your counterpart.

ACT II

SCENE I

In this scene the characters are comic and full of valour, sympathetic and humourous as what seemed a tragedy is turning into a comedy. Mark you, the Sole sufferer is the patient throughout the whole play. It is evident that all his relations and acquaintants are affected and confused by false rummour from the society. This brings complications and misunderstanding to those who are not aware of the happenings. The patient is very sensitive to what actually happens. He compared what is happening with his past experiences and makes his judgement. The whole issue is peculiar but patient is encouraged by some good friends to take courage.

Tipuan: (Comes in in a beautiful coat singing and is followed by his American girl. The girl speaks some broken Menka dialect.)

Girl: (Come round demonstrating how she will handle her cutlery at meal time.) This is the way I handle my cultery (speaks as if she is whispering. Girl in shadowy form.)

Patient: (Pays no heed to such actions.
Patient notices Tipuan at the other side of the house having the same meals with him. [102])

Demon Tipuan: Now, you know that whatever you think you drink or eat here in this house you are not doing so alone but with people you cannot see them.
(Tipuan goes under the floor into his house and patient notices a bright and blue parlour illuminated by blue lights. He also sees a strange type of fowl).

Patient: (Left a lone in thoughts of a series of mysterious events. He speaks to himself aloud.)
This is like a dagger to my heart while people should speak broken Menka expressions. I see no cause to do this. Even if this has a future meaning, why should the language be immoral?
Everything relates to sex, slander and gossip [103]. The greatest enemies in an up to date society. This should really give me much food for thought.
I am sure enough, this occurence is an artful trick performed by some personalities to suffer me for nothing but for their own selfish aims. Murderers are often arrested and questioned. Thieves and other evil doers in the society punished and some go gay. What is the point in these series of events without even a soul around to cool one's mind, from various thoughts imposed into him by actions of people, through aweful dreams, words and shadows. Is this a subversive movement or this happens in everyone's life time?
The different forms, appearances of persons are therefore presented by the people of the locality to exhibit their spiritualism over human beings. Some people must have transformed themselves into such figures especially figures of those I know. It is therefore an attempt to make me suspicious of everyone wherever I go [104]. If the figures are really dead spirits, the people concerned must have invoked them in order to know more about me and those I know.

ACT II

SCENE II

Arrival of Rev. Fr. Sullivan, Rose Gana and Bridget Awasum From London

Fr. Sullivan: (In an invisible form speaking on my head. He introduces himself and the girls and all of them went through me.) I have come along from Britain with the girls I told you yesterday. They are Rose Gana and Bridget Awasum.

Rose Gana: (Introduces herself before her journey through my body.) I am Rose Gana speaking to you. I have been told that you are ill and have therefore followed Father Sullivan to come and see you.

Bridget Awasum: (Introduces herself to patient.)
I am Bridget Awasum speaking to you. I have come here to see you because I heard that you are ill. It is really difficult in many places to speak to someone whom people dislike for personal reasons. So this form in which we are is applicable in some places, and is the only possible way in which we can come to you. (Patient is quite familiar with the two girls but as he cannot see them he is in doubt.)

Bridget Awasum: (Asks patient to prepare for a snap shot.)
Get ready for a snap shot. (She leaves patient and soon he hears her speaking at the opposite wall.)
Are you ready? Steady, Steady. (Patient sees flash of light.)
It is alright, (she says.)
I will tell you a message to deliver to someone in a hilly village in Bamenda.

The three Visitors: (One speaking.) Goodbye. We are going away now and in three hours time we shall be in London. (The three visitors return back. There is some disturbance on the road caused by some Cameroonians.)

Father Sullivan: There is some trouble on the way caused by some Cameroonians. I cannot go without these girls. I have come back to rinforce myself with some medicine from some English men who are around before leaving finally at about three o' clock the next morning.

An Orator: (A typical Rural Menka man full of knowledge of the present society, experienced and fluent in speaking his native tongue.)

Patient: (Sitting down in a lonely world dominated by spirits. He pictures above him by the side of the wall, someone swimming in a horizontal manner. Actually he is stretching his legs and his hands rhythmically. It appears he is fixed to the spot and can push himself to any direction with ease. Patient recognises him by voice; probably Mr. Mpong. He makes a speech in vernacula.)

M p o n g : (Speaking in unison with the movement.) It is good to be friendly. Good friends should love themselves and have an out-going concern for one another. The society, the world all over will be dull if people are not friendly. A miracle has brought different people of the world together. Although the oceans, culture and distance divide us; yet people of different countries have found that there is necessity to communicate with other distant places. This relationship has brought about peace, encourage people to co-operate and advance in knowledge with rich ideas. We have been to Mr. Vincent Abang, Tiko, and we are here now. It is because we have the interest to see you. As I am speaking, I am heard everywhere in this town. We have been to many places in the federated State of West Cameroon. We shall enter the Prime Minister and speak to him "only" in our vernacula.
There is a witchcraft called "Nyamgzah" by which we can go to any place. We have had several encounters on the road with Kumba people. We understand any language when we are in this form.
(The scene closes in a fight between patient's father and Mr. Elonge.)

M r . E l o n g e : (He is guarded by some animals like girraffs, he shoots out a very long tooth from his mouth.)

F a t h e r : (Changing into many forms, first the snake, then snake pouring out fire from its mouth, the snake defending itself with shields and so on. In this instance he is building a rocky house for protection and is aided by Mr. Tandu.)

M o t h e r : (Mother is also attacked in this struggle but the inquisitor is warned and mother goes off.)

ACT II SCENE III

D o c t o r : (The shadow of Doctor Lantum steps in and assumes the position of the first person who made a speech formerly. He repeats what he did but makes no speech.)

S o l d i e r : (The house in which patient lives is a twin house. In the neighbouring section is a soldier who has come to spend sometime with his girl friend.)

P a t i e n t S i t t i n g d o w n : (Notices the soldier's shadow piercing through a door closed totally for entry. The shadow sits on the table and makes no noise. In a while the two figures vanish.)

D e m o n T i p u a n : (Shouting in annoyance.)
Leave this parlour and go to your bedroom. By tomorrow you should leave this place and go somewhere.

P a t i e n t : (Insists and sits down quietly.)

T i p u a n : (Shouts with irritating voice.
This time, he is speaking under patients feet.)
I say again leave this room and go to your bedroom.
Many people are coming here for a meeting.

Patient: (Moves away amazed. He lies in his bed and falls into a sleep. After sometime he feels a streaming movement like that of maggots in his bed. Patient takes up his head and listens.)

Conny Van Zanten: (European accent, speaks fluently. Should be invisible, warns patient to go as already said.) You will like to learn more from me. After our stay in Bamenda we shall be studying in London hospital with you. I will teach you some Dutch.

Mathias Ntar: (Delegated by Rev. Fr. Sullivan.)
I am delegated by Father Sullivan to speak to you. Get some money and go to Tiko and consult Doctor Lantum.

Patient: (Conscious of last night's warning does not hesitate. He advises his junior brother to stay in the house until he returns. He boards a taxi for Tiko without delay.)

People: (Here some disorderly invisible group of persons should be speaking and advising the patient.)

Patient: (In disgust, worried by voices speaking under his laps as he sits down. Some speaking pidgin, some English and other his vernacula.)

Voice: (Menacing advice through the window which enters patient's ears in the form of breeze.)

Akam: We are here protecting you. If we go away some people may take away your life. (Speaking under patient's seat.)

Spirits: Look at the front window of the taxi, and you will see the picture of Doctor Lantum.

Patient: (On looking, sees a bright picture of the Doctor.)

Speaking to Himself: (He is at Tiko in Doctor's house, meets Doctor's wife and some women. Here patient should speak aloud.)
Is this not the picture I saw on the window of the taxi I boarded? [105]
(He looks at the picture surprisingly. He is already in Doctor Lantum's house.)

Patient: (A knock at the door.)

Mrs. Lantum: Come in.

Mrs. Lantum: Good evening, Mr. Tanka. You are from....

Patient: From Kumba.

Mrs. Lantum: What can I do for you?

Patient: I have come to consult the Doctor.

Mrs. Lantum: Yes, you look quite pale (speaks as though she has had a foreknowledge of my illness.) He is still at work in the hospital. Do you want private consultation?

Patient: It is too late for me to see him in the office. So I think it is better to consult him privately.

Mrs. Lantum: Sitdown and wait for him. He will soon come. What brand will you take?

Patient: (Speaks hesitatingly.) I will take any.

Mrs. Lantum :(Offers a bottle of beer and a glass to patient.)

Patient: Thank you madam. (He opens the beer and drinks it gradually.)

Doctor Lantum: (Foot steps up the stairs, walks elegantly into the house.)

Patient: (Stands up, and greets him) Good evening, Sir.

Doctor Lantum: Good evening.
(Walks to his seat.)

Mrs. Lantum: This is Mr. Tanka, a clerk in the Education Dept. He is at the moment working in the Education office, Kumba. He has come to consult you.

Doctor Lantum: (Turning in his seat and facing the patient.)
Yes, what can I do for you? You are who again?

Patient: I am Benedict N. Tanka. I know you very well. You used to teach us biology in Sasse and I had often seen you on holidays while you were still in the University.

Doctor Lantum: What is your complaint?

Patient: Yesterday evening, at 8 p.m. in my house, I heard a mysterious command and unconsciously obeyed it but failed to see who made the mysterious command.

Doctor Lantum: What was the command?

Patient: "The Prime Minister has asked you to walk to the door, stand on your heels, look to the left and right and you will see a girl by your window named Angela Ndefru," That was the command.

Doctor: Did you see the Girl?

Patient: I did not see any person at all.

Doctor: Is that all?

Patient: No. After meditating for a long time, I went to bed confused. In the night, I felt a movement inside my body, acute and piercing my flesh like a needle. Then a voice said, "I am Mr. Andela, Secretary to the Prime Minister speaking to you. When I speak do not speak but only listen to me. I am here with Doctor Lantum. Your nerves are very strong and it is very difficult for anyone to go through." Later on I recognised two shadows by my bed side. A minute later, something like an insect spoke on my head. Saying "another Doctor has entered you" and at this I felt a scraping and painful movement around the inside part of my waist, continuing, the spirit says "It is Doctor Nasah. They have all come to examine you."

Doctor: Go home and report to me tomorrow in the hospital at 8 a.m. Have you a place to sleep here in Tiko? (He goes off to the dinning table with his wife).

Patient: I have some of my country boys here but I will like to spend my night at Mutengene.

Patient: (Continues to drink his beer. He bids good night to Doctor and wife and walks out of the house.
He comes to a road junction and boards a taxi for Mutengene. He alights from the taxi and goes to Betty's residence, finds door locked. He tries to open the door but it is difficult.)

Patient: (Enquiring a neighbour of Betty's whereabouts.) Where is Betty?

Teacher: She is gone to Soppo for holiday and will be back next Wednesday.

Patient: Thank you for your information. Good night.
(He gets another taxi for Bolyfamba C. D. C. camp. There he takes shelter with relatives and he tells them of his trouble. It sounds very ambiguous to everyone.)

Patient: (The following morning he hears a lady's voice whispering under his feet. One of his father's wifes probably speaking. Mother of his hostess.)

Mama Yafuan: Here is your inlaw. You can always come here when you are in difficulty. Can you not ask him to give you something? (She continues to speak to patient on his way and leads him to Tiko.)

Patient: (Boards a Government landrover for Tiko. He is pricked and confused within and without by the mysterious voices. He cannot listen or think of any other thing but the voices. He is exhausted and almost sweating because of the pressure of pains in his body and the noises. Watch falls off from his hand and he takes no notice of this until after he has left the landrover. He looks at his hand, sighs and goes off to the hospital.)

Patient: (Walking into the clerk's office.)
Good morning, please. Where can I pay the consultation fee?

Clerk: Go to the clerk on that table (pointing to the clark.)

Patient: Good morning.

Clerk: Good morning.

Patient: I want to pay consultation fee in order to see the Doctor.
(He hands money to clerk and issues a receipt.)

Patient: (Goes to the counter clerk for a hospital card.)

Counter Clerk: Where is your receipt?

Patient: Here it is.

Counter Clerk: (Looks at it and issues a hospital card to patient.)

Patient: (Walking into the Dr.'s consulting room and sees but a lady Doctor.) Good morning, Doctor.

Doctor: Good morning. What is your complain?

Patient: Two days ago at about 8 p.m. I heard a command in my house and unconsciously obeyedit. I saw no person who made the noise and was dumb-founded and perplexed for the whole time. The next morning, I heard some voices telling me this and that in my house, on the way and inside the church. Really everywhere I was mercilessly tormented. In the night till the next morning, I felt the most painful movement and prickings in my head and in my whole body. It was burning like fire and something dropping from the walls of my stomach and chest and these seemed to be like blood and water.

Doctor: Is that all?

Patient: Yes

Doctor: (Prescribes medicine.)

Patient: (Receives treatment and later goes to the senior medical officer.)

Patient: I have consulted the lady Doctor and have received some treatment.

Doctor: Let me see your card.

Patient: (Hands the card to him and he glances through. He prescribes more medicine and asks me to go for it.)

Doctor: Go and take this medicine befor you come.

Patient: (Goes for the medicine.)

Doctor: Have you got your tablets?

Patient: Yes, sir.

Doctor: Sit down. Where do you work and who is your head of Dept?

Patient: I work in Education Officer, Kumba and my head of Dept. is Director of Education.

Doctor: Are you in agreement with your boss? Does he like you?

Patient: I cannot say exactly because what I may consider good may be bad to him. He is someone who is easily annoyed and he looks a talkertive person.

Doctor: For how long have you been working without leave?

Patient: About three years.

Doctor: How old are you and what is your ambition?

Patient: I am 26 years old and I read for the G. C. E. examination. [106]

Doctor: I am recommending to your Director that you go on two months sick leave to treat yourself. (He drafts two letters and passes them for typing.) You will take these along with you, hand one to your head of Dept. and the other you will give to the medical officer of Acha Tugi hospital in Gwofon.
You will endeavour to report to me after your treatment with a medical report. You must be very careful with your health and lastly I recommend that you buy medicine from the chemist too to reduce the tension of illness in you.

Patient:(Receives letters and thanks the Doctor.)

Patient: Good morning, Sir.

Director: Good morning, Tanka, what do you want?

Patient: Here is a letter from the Doctor, General Hospital Tiko, approving that I should go to Acha Tugi for treatment.

Director: (Takes letter and reads.)But this is not from a Government medical officer.

Patient: The Government medical officer failed to discover my illness.

Director: Alright you can go.

Patient: (Walks out of the office thanking Director. He boards, a taxi for Kumba.)

ACT III SCENE IV

The result of the warning comes out in this scene. Patient and brother abandon house and go off to Bamenda.

Patient: (Arriving from Tiko and finding the compound so quiet. The doors all locked and old foot prints at the door. It was exactly 7. 30 and on opening the door he finds a lamp glowing on the table.)

Patient: (Speaking to himself.)
It is too late for someone to be out now. This fellow is not used to go to places. What must be wrong with him? The lamp has been lighted and it is burning on the table. Does it therefore mean it was lighted two days ago? (It is exactly nine o'clock and he is weary and has to sleep. Philip comes in the next day.)

Patient: Philip, where did you sleep?

Philip: In the town.

Patient: Who told you to go there and for heaven's sake with whom were you spending your time?

Philip: I went there with Miss Rose Enow.

Patient: Why did you have to accompany her? You have never been doing that in the past.

Philip: The first daughter of our neighbour died yesterday.

Patient: What caused her death? Before I left she was quite well.

Philip: A snake beat her the night you left for Tiko. She was taken to the hospital and the following morning, she died. I had to go to the town because Miss Enow asked me to go with her and secondly I was afraid to be here alone.

Patient: I am very ill and I must go to Acha Tugi hospital for treatment. After this, I will also like to consult a native Doctor, at home [107]. I do not know how long I shall be in the hospital. Consequently I can't let you to be here alone. You must go with me and at Bamenda I shall let you go home while I go to the hospital, meanwhile after your holiday you should tell Simon to find a place for you in R. C. M. School Widekum. You should inform parents that I am at Acha for treatment. Don't tell them that I am seriously ill.
I am leaving you now, make sure you greet everyone for me.

Patient: Good morning, Sir.
Here is a letter from Doctor Lantum, C. D. C. hospital Tiko.

Doctor Schwarz: (Tall, simple, good mannered man, receives letter, opens and reads it.)
Oh yes, I know Doctor Lantum. (He reads the diagnosis of my illness. He takes me to a waiting room. On the table are a pile of pictures of strange flowers for me [108]).
Sit down on this chair. Here are some pictures. You have to study them. I shall be coming round for a test. (The 'I' here is ironical because the person to come will be a 'she' the Doctor's wife who is also a Doctor. He walks out.).

Patient: (Looks at different shapes of the pictures. In fact, he thought the pictures were some bones of the vetebral column. All the time he compares them with the different bones of this column.)

A lady Doctor: Good morning. Have you finished studying these pictures?

Patient: I do not seem to understand the pictures. I do not know what they represent.

Doctor: You have got to say anything about them. I am going to write down all what you can say about each picture.

Patient: (Describes to the Doctor his knowledge of the pictures.)

Doctor: That is alright. (She goes out with a copy of the description for the result. Patient is later admitted as an out patient.)

Doctor: (Prescribes medicine, six strong injections and some tablets.) You will take these injections in six days time. You will be reporting here every day. Take the injections to the injection room.

Patient: I have been asked to give this to you.

Nurse: (Receives injections and administers one.) Go and come tomorrow. (Patient walks out. It is just 5 o'clock. He catches taxi for Bamenda. He is weakened by the injection, and this is marked by a series of uncontrolled yawning, and very high fever. He hears voices speaking from above, he sights some figure in white apparel. Arrives Bamenda at 8 p.m. but is so weak and cannot go to his lodging house. Fortunately for him, he recognises an old school mate from his voice and asks him to assist him.) I cannot walk at all. I am so weak to go to Joe's house. My eyes are weak and my senses weak. I don't even know the direction to his house now. Can you please lead me to your house to spend this night only with you? I will go to him tomorrow.

Friend: (Shows willingness and kindness. He leads patient to his house.)

Patient: I am so cool and I will like to bath myself at a fire.

Friend: (Makes a big fire). You will have to take a bath.

Patient: (Takes a bath and goes back to the fire side. Finds difficulty in taking a meal. He sleeps with hunger.)

Friend: (Leads him to a bare bamboo bed. Patient goes to bed but finds it difficult to sleep. A night of dreams.)

Patient: (At day dawn he gets ready and asks friend to lead him to Joe.)

Joe: Ben, welcome, how is your health?

Patient: I am seriously ill. I arrived here yesterday but was unable to reach the house. But for this friend, I would have slept on the road side. (On saying this he sits on a bench in the bank).

Joe: (Hurries up to the Driver.) Can you please take this patient to my house? He cannot travel. (Driver takes patient to the house. Patient goes to bed at once.)

Patient: (Finds difficulty to breath or sleep.)

Joe Returns from Work

Joe: Get up and take some food.

Patient: (Struggles out of bed. Yawns every blessed second and finds difficulty in eating. Cannot chew the food as he yawns every time.) Joe, I am alright. I am really hungry but find it difficult to eat.

Period of (convalescent) Recovering.

For three weeks, patient remains in bed receiving treatment during which time his brothers visited him and as the Doctor finds him a little improved, he releases him and sends a letter for Dr. Lantum.

Brother: The next news about your illness stroke us with great anxiety and pity and our mother and some others were almost weeping. Really, it beats our imagination as we are ignorant of the nature of illness. Father would have come here with me but as he found Philip with me, he told me to come and verify if there is any improvement.

Patient: I dare say that you would not take it serious; for my health is a little bit improved and tell exactly what I am telling you to our parents so that they shouldn't have any fear. I am going to be here for one week again and I will make sure that I report to our parents before I go back to my station. I pray that you tender my sincere regards to everyone. I wish you a safe journey home. (At this they shake hands and off they went. Patient pays his last visit to the Doctor.)

Patient: Good morning, Doctor.

Doctor: Good morning Mr. Tanka. How is your health?

Patient: I feel a little bit better than before.

Doctor: Good, and have you finished all the medicine and the injections?

Patient: Yes Doctor, everything finished two days ago.

Doctor: What will you want me do for you now?

Patient: I will like to go back to my Station. But first of all, I must see my parents before I go back and secondly Doctor Lantum asked me to make sure that I receive a medical report from you before I leave for Kumba and this report must be presented to him for his scrutiny.

Doctor: Alright. Sit down and wait for the letter.

The Report: The M.O., Doctor Lantum, Tiko.

Dear Sir,

We have seen your patient, Mr. B. Tanka (Your ref. TH/WC 8.4.18) on 22/4, 23/4 and 7/5/68.
Diagnosis: Confirmed, Schizophrenia, paranoide.
Other Results: Hgb 87% Microfiloria in skin-snip posRohrschach's psychodiagnostic: not very pathological.

Treatment: Administered: Personal interviews and psycholepticum per injectionem resulted into a relaxing sleeping-course during 1 week (had at home by dispenser,) at final consultation: Taractan 25 mg t.d.s. Sandoxal: 1 or 2 tabs. at bed time. Subjectively he feels " a bit better. " Main complaint the sleeplessness. We advised him to postpone his plans with G. C. E. etc. Paranoid ideas now not openly admitted but referred to dreams.
Patient deposited a note full of dreams; on request we could send it in.

Yours

Dr. Schwarz, M.O.

Take this letter to the Doctor. Have you written an account of more dreams as I told you?

Patient: No Doctor. I thought that the ones I gave you were sufficient for the purpose.

Doctor: Yes, they are but I thought that you have brought more. Alright Mr. Tanka, I wish you well and safe journey home. (Doctor shakes hand with him and off he goes.)

Patient reports to Parents:

Father: Welcome my son. I have heard all types of stories about your health. I therefore sent your brother to come and visit you and bring back news to me of your condition of health.

Patient: Many people tell me that my parents are the cause of my illness, [109] but I refuse to admit what they told me because I know that my parents cannot have any ill feelings about me.

Father: What do I want from you that I cannot ask you in words? But to suffer you indirectly? Are you God to know my thoughts? The evil people who are accusing your parents must be responsible for this. You can't expect a father to give a stone nor a serpent to his son, that needs a piece of bread or a fish. God will eventually reward these Wicked men. I pray that the medicines you have taken should improve your health [110]. The time is too short for me to call a native Doctor for you but I promise to do this when you come here next time. You should return home for treatment if your health continues to fall back into its old condition. (Parents see off Patient.)

The snake at 11 p.m.

(Snake ambushes under patient's pillows in readiness to bite. Patient lies in bed without knowing. He is tantalised by a hissing sound coming under the pillow. He raised up his head instantly and the snake stands up erect ready to bite. At the sight of a matchet and a club in patient's hands, snake glides off quickly [111]. Patient is left alone in thoughts shivering with a panting heart. At day dawn he leaves for Tiko.)

Patient: Good morning, Doctor.

Doctor: Good morning. Have you returned from Acha Tugi?

Patient: Yes, Doctor.

Doctor: I hope your health is quite improved.

Patient: It is just a little bit but the tension is not as great as it was before.

Doctor: I will have to prescribe more medicine for you and now what else will you like me to do for you?

Patient: I am not at all happy with the environments and the society in which I live, I suggest that I leave the locality.

Doctor Recommends Transfer: [112]

Body of Letter: "I am happy to release Mr. Tanka now to you. He is now much improved and can resume work.
But as he has great propensity for relapsing into his old condition, I am here recommending that he should be removed from environments that are likely to precipitate his old condition. Bamenda and Buea are likely to constitute favourable environments for his health considering the physical and social climate. But wherever he resumes, I would further recommend that he will be put on light duty i. e. duty free of many intellectual challenges and exacting contemplation, for at least one month."

Dr. D. Lantum: But wherever you go on transfer be very careful with yourself and buy medicine from the chemists. If you are transferred to Buea endeavour to consult me from time to time but if you are transferred to Bamenda you will be going to Acha Tugi for consultation. (Patient goes on transfer to the Work in Gowfon. He sees no difference between his new station and the old. Instead things got worsened. He tells his Doctors everything.)

Patient receiving treatment in his home town:

Native Doctor: It is the evil spirit that is troubling you. Some people whom you know dislike you have poisened you [113]. This may be because of your work or because of "Women affairs." I am going to give you this medicine and it will help you. -
(The treatment lasted for only three days and it was necessary to seek some medical attention before returning to work. All my vacation were spent at Gwofon. There was no difference here too. Everything was as usual. The few friends here Mr. Shu, the Agric Officer, Mr. Ntoko, the Post Master were of great help to me. Story is narrated to them.)

Mr. Shu: Mr. Ben. Your story is somewhat peculiar and mysterious to me and I see that you have received the worst of punishment so far. You look pale and weak. You seem to think so much and you have very little sleep. As you are here you must not only concern yourself with medical treatment, you see. I will like to suggest that you also seek the native Doctors for consultation too.

Patient: This I have already started in my native home before coming here. You can see so many marks and wounds which the native Doctor made [114]. All I want is a quick recovery and I don't care if I sell all my little property just to get well.

Mr. Shu: Exactly. Your good health counts first. When you are well you will buy more.

Mr. Ntoko: Your story is very touching to everyone of us and I dare not say much about it but I believe that drugs will make you feel well within a short time [115].

Patient: (Shows feelings of appreciation at the advice and decides to have a thorough medical examination to know more about his health before resuming duty. The hospital is about fourteen miles away from the station. Just about 4 hours trek.)

Patient: Good morning Doctor.

Doctor: Good morning, Mr. Tanka. How are you now?

Patient: There is nothing quite different about my health. It is just the same as it was after my last treatment here but the voices and dreams I told you of seem to have worsened the condition. Doctor Lantum has recommended that I should come here and he is gone to overseas for further studies. As I have to resume duty here, I think it wise to consult the Doctor for a medical check up before I start duty, I have been transferred to work in Gwofon here but unfortunately there is no office here for our Dept. But I have been asked by my officer to bring all my property to Gwofon.

Doctor: Go and sit near the X-ray room and I shall come and attend to you.

Patient: (Walks out of the consulting room and take seat at the corridor near the X-ray room.)

Doctor: (Enters the room, switched off lights and asks patient to strip off all his clothes except his pant.)
Come nearer, stand erect. Yes, everything is finished. Go and wait for the results.(Doctor gives report after one hours time.)

Doctor: (Fills the report.)
The miraculous voices, movement in your body and the dreams have resulted to the break down of your nervous system. It is now quite normal but I am warning you to be very careful with yourself as this may likely occur again. You know what this organ does to your body and when you become unreasonable you are regarded as a mad man.
(After a period of 1 1/2 months at Gwofon patient moves to Bamenda. He was already familiar with the new office and the staff but some of the Staff use to put up a contenance of stern commandment which spoke very much about the persons. Patient does not hesitate in his usual ill-health mood to make a report to the S.S.P. [116])

Patient: Good morning, Sir.
I am now working here. I was sent here as a result of ill-health. First of all I have been in Gwofon and now I am here.

S.S.P.: What is wrong with you?

Patient: Tells his story.

S.S.P.: This is a strange thing to me.
You should be very careful with yourself. Tell this to your boss so that you are not treated in the wrong way.

Patient: (Reporting to boss the S. S. P. ' advice.)

Please sir, I have already informed you about my health and you have read letters about it from the Doctor. I have just been to the S. S. P. and have told him everything about it. He has asked me to tell you to inform everyone in this office not to offend me.

Period of Convalescence

(Father sends two girls [117] to comfort and nurse patient with a letter. Patient reads letter carefully.)

Dear Son,

Since you left me, I have not been very happy at all especially when I viewed the critical situation of your health and the strange type of illness you described to me.

Although you said that staying with a helper incurs much expenditure, I view this with a most sympathetic heart and thought it wise to send you these children to be with you until your health improves. We are all well at home.

I wish you God's blessing.

I am your loving father,

Papa Nta.

(Patient speaking happily to his first visitors since his three months stay in Bamenda.)

Why did you have to wait until now? I told you to follow me after a few weeks but you over stayed.

Bridget: Mother was not quite well and secondly I had a sore on my leg and hence I could not keep to your suggestion.

Patient: How is she now and everyone else? Did you also go to my father before coming here?

Bridget: Mother is improving now or else I should not have come here. I went to grandfather a week before coming. He has not told you anything very special but has asked me to convey his greetings to you.

Patient: You are also welcome to my new station. How is home and everything else?

Florence: Home is good and everyone is well. But we have not been happy to hear of your illness. I couldn't just persevere.

Patient: Do you think the two of you will cure me in a short time? How shall you people stay here when I shall be going to see my medicine people?

Florence: We can stay here as you have been spending plenty of money for the illness.

Patient: Will you not be afraid to be here alone as you have not been here before?

Florence: Why should we be afraid? Are they not people living here?

Patient: Bridget, what do you say about this?

Bridget: I hold fast to what my friend has just said. Nothing can happen to us here.

Patient: Good God has sent me my nurses to be nursing me in my sick bed.

Station Workers Around the Police Office

Here any aweful sounds relating to patient's health, relatives and friends should be made. e.g.
"Call me clerk mama; "
"Call me clerk sasa, the jooly"
"Enong yi Muo yiyi Wuequit, Ye puh buoh. "
"Our Lourdes, Our Lourdes, "
"Anastah, Ntar. " etc.
Romance in sounds through the nose and other catch-words such as "Ah gendah gah" Buea, Winka, Atichequeh.
"Agendah Ya bili muah"

Patient:(Interpreted these sounds.)
These sounds are meaningless to me [118]. Any average man who has anything to tell me should walk up straight and speak his mind on me. I see no reason why I am constandly being put into imoral, rebellious thoughts and made to reflect on the past. Such thoughts are not good and they portray a darkimage of my character. Worst of all, thoughts are easily inducted by others [118], what is all this to me?
(Patient tells this to the Doctor.)

Doctor: Your story is very strange. I must tell you that the voices are not from people but the reflection of your own thoughts. These come back to you in the form of sounds [119].

Patient: Please, Sir, I have experienced this several times. I do not see why the sounds should be made everywhere I go? Usually I hear some names I have not thought of. Yesterday for an example I heard some and when I asked my neighbour, they told me that they also heard it. I do not mean that people should not shout or say anything. But they assasinate my thoughts with impure sounds usually relating to my family men and some friends.

Doctor: It is an illness and it takes a long time before it is treated. However, I am recommending that you rest in bed for one month and you must be reporting to me every Tuesday.(After three weeks patient tells Doctor that there was no improvement and that the noises were still being made. He suggests that he could seek the attention of a native Doctor.)

Doctor: You must see him and bring me his findings and I will know what to do [120].

Patient: I fell ill at Kumba before I was sent here. I have been receiving medical attention and although there is little improvement I find it necessary to consult a native Doctor because I see that my illness is somewhat very unatural.

Native Doctor: What happened to you?

Patient: I heard a command in my house and obey it. I saw no person who made the command. I also felt some movement within my body and at the same time some people were speaking in my body.

Native Doctor: Come nearer to me. Open your right hand palm. (He looks at it, touched a table here and there and said certain words.)

Patient: (Is very careful and looks at the native Doctor and his actions. Doctor chews some medicine and each time he discovers something from his spirits he informs patient.)

Native Doctor: Your parents have nothing in heart about you. You were not in agreement with your boss in the office. A meeting was held and a lady was delagated to wrought some spell on you [113]. It is difficult for me to call the name of the person because the poison was put in you by a spirit. If it was given to you in drink or food I will be able to call his name.

Patient: Was it the poison that was speaking in my body? And right now I feel pains in my stomach and all over my body.

Native Doctor: Yes, it is the ailment that is working in you. You have really overcome its effects with medical drugs without which you would have died [121]. But you should not fear anything again. I will give you some medicine and you should continue to take the medicine from the chemists.

Patient: I saw many shadows in my house. Saw some men who died many years ago. Some were my late relatives and others were shadows of people 'alive'.

Native Doctor: Yes this is an easy thing. They did this to deceive you. The spirits can take any form. The spirits that represented your family men and friends were put in front to deceive you. You did not see the evil spirits. For sake of formality I will like you to make a small feast to your people.
Do not keep your native customs aside. Ordinary people did this not your parents. You will have to pay 2,000 for the drugs I will give you. (Patient pays bill to Doctor, gives goodbye and goes home. He takes drugs for a week but saw no improvement.)

Patient Reports to Doctor (Medical)

I received some drugs from a native Doctor and have been taking this for a whole week but it has been of no avail to me. I will like to go to my home place for another consultation to a native Doctor and also to Oku.
These are the last two places I must go to.

Doctor Recommends Leave

(Issues a letter recommanding six weeks leave.) Report to me after consulting the native Doctors. (Patient goes home, prepares to live next morning for Nso. The arrival of Cousin Anastasia and Mr. Abang.)

Patient: (Schedules cousin to stay until his return.) Oh! at last you have come just on the eve of my departure to Oku for medical attention. God is really with me. Did you get the information by your spirits as others get information from my thoughts?

Cousin: No. I saw your letter but I could not come early because my husband could not allow me. But last night I told him that I must come today and that is why I am here. The story of spirits' is strange to me.

Mr. William: My own mission is quite different. I have come here to see my boss, the supervisor, about my school and to buy some School equipment too.

Cousin: When will you come back as you are so much in haste?

Patient: I do not know. This is a decision to be taken at Oku.

Mr. William: I am sure there is very little time for us for discussion. I thought that the evening and the whole of our stay here will be very useful in your presence. I am sorry as you are going away.
(Patient is seen off by cousin for Oku.
Patient arrives Nso and goes to legal Dept.)

Patient: Where is Mr. Gabriel Takwon?

Friend: Go to the extreme door and you will get him in the office.
(Gabriel is found in the office.)

Gabriel: You are welcomed. What has brought you here?

Patient: Illness has brought me here. I am going to Oku but I feel that I must see you before I go.

Gabriel: I have heard of your illness and I do not know how this come to happen. Let us go to the house before you go.

Patient: How far is it from here to Oku?

Gabriel: It is about 17-18 miles. The road is motorable, but only on Oku market days i.e. once in the week. The market will be on Monday. Exactly three days from today.

Patient: I can't wait here for up to three days. It is just one thirty now and I must reach there today. I don't care if anything happen to me on the way.

Gabriel: Its so hot and you look tired. We must go to the house for lunch before you go. What will you like to drink?

Patient: I will like to take a small guinness stout.

Cousin: (Rejoicing runs forward to receive patient.) Welcome. How is Bamenda and home?

Patient: Bamenda and home are fine except me. How is your baby?

Cousin: Baby is well. I am happy to see you. It is long time since I saw you. Almost three years ago.

Patient: Hurry with the meal. I do not want to waste time here. Also get some kola nuts for me. I hear that there is very little food there.

Patient: (Takes a little of the meal and goes off. He is led some distance off by the friends. The long trek of 12 miles. Car picks patient at about 5 p.m.)

Patient: (Stopping car.)

Driver: Where are you going to?

Patient: I am going to Oku.

Driver: Will you pay 300 francs?

Patient: Wonderful, 300 francs for only 7 miles?

Driver: Yes, if you do not, I will go.

Patient: It is getting dark. I will pay 150 francs.

Driver: (Glides off with car but stops again after a few yards.)
Come and pay the money.

Patient: (Rushes up to the car.
He gets in and the car started off.
In the car a gentleman, Mr. James Ndikaka says the native Doctor is his brother and he is staying there in "small London" [122] 4 miles away from Oku town.)

Ndikaka and Patient: (Take some drink in an inn.)

Native Doctor: (Arriving Ndikaka introduces me to native Doctor. An aged, medium height, dark in complexion man who spoke no language other than his dialect. His house is full of people. Has a large compound with many women and grand children. He asks me of my mission. Illness, patient narrated. He is in grief (sister died) and asks an attendant to lead patient to a house for the night.)

Patient: I have a message for your daughter from my friend. As you have assured me. She will come on Sunday.

Ndikaka: Yes, we shall meet on Sunday and surely I will ask her to see you here.
(On Sunday neither of them turned up.)

Native Doctor: (Calls patient.)
Strip up your vests, your glasses, your cap and leave only your trousers. Come nearer and sit on this chair. (This is an interpretation of

the native Doctor by his interpreter). Native Doctor sits on one side of the door, his interpreter on the other and patient in the middle. Native Doctor says certain things in his language [123].

Interpreter: (Holding a fresh plantain leaf in his hand. He explains in pidgin English what the native doctor says.)
You are in love with a certain lady and many people jealous you. They do not like that you make love [124] with that girl. That is the whole thing about it.

Patient: What then shall I do?

Doctor: You cannot do anything. But I am going to give you some drugs to drink and some to take home. This will help and cure you.

Patient: Should I discontinue friendship with the girl?

Native Doctor: No. Why should you?
But you will bring along with you this evening, the sum of 17,000 francs for the medicine I will give you.

Patient: I will pay you 8,000 francs.

Native Doctor: I will only accept it because you are just a new man here. Go and sleep and tomorrow you will receive your drugs and go home since you don't want to stay here again.
(Remember injection liquid.)
(Patient receives some "injection liquid" which sets him rolling several times unconsciously [125]).

Patient: (Brings bill next morning, and receives some medicine from the native Doctor.)

Native Doctor: (In a hideous place under tree outside the house administers treatment.)

Native Doctor: (Makes a mighty cut at the back of patient's neck, on his forehead and on his right foot and put in some medicine.) You have to slap this stone with your left hand palm once only, otherwise you will kill someone on attempting to slap him.
(Patient slaps stone as he is bidden to do so.
Native Doctor says certain things in his dialect, lastly he asks patient to repeat some sentences.)
I believe in God and with him everything is possible. This medicine which I have taken will cure me through the power of God. (Patient repeats the words of the Native Doctor.)

Native Doctor: Take these small sticks (five in number) and drop them in the big stream over which a bridge crosses. Drop them on the downwards side and do not look at them while dropping. When dropping them say that I believe in God and trough his power this medicine will cure me.
(Patient performs action and crosses bridge. A few yards off, he is met by Ndikaka [126].)

Patient and Ndikaka: (Meet at an inn again in Oku for some drink. Farewell wish to each other. Patient passes home for treatment. At home the best drugs were received and the symptoms were almost reduced.)

Native Doctor: This is the second time I am treating you. I will treat you in three rounds. So one round is remaining, that is the last stage of my treatment. I have already told you everything about your illness.

Patient to Doctor Muna [127]:
I have been to Oku and to Menka, my home place. The medicines I received at home helped me a great deal. Here too there was very little noise. In fact, the first time I went home there was no noise at all but this time it was surprising to me when I heard some noise too, and the same as elsewhere but I improved in health. I fear to stay here long because conditions will soon go bad, I am pleading that I be moved from this place to the South. I saw Doctor Schwarz yesterday in the market and I told him everything and he suggested it worth while for me to go down immediately and live in good condition.

Doctor: Do you think Buea is better than this place? You will get the same noise everywhere. However, I will recommend that you go down to Buea.

Letter of Recommendation: General Hospital Bamenda.

The S.E.O. Bamenda. (Senior Education Officer.)

We have been following Mr. Tanka Medically since August 22nd 1969 and have noted considerable improvement in his condition. I recommend that he should return to work, be placed on light duty that does not require exactness and too much concentration, and be observed for 3 months. I cannot rule out the possibility of relapse in this case. Buea now appears to be an untried but possibly favourable environment for him to work.

Thank you.

Doctor Muna, Medical Officer.

Patient: (Hands Recommendation to Director.)

Director: Go and sit down I will pass it to the Establishment Secretary, and ask him to send you to a different Department as there is no room for you here.

Establishment Secretary: (Replies saying that thorough medical attention should be sought.)

Director Replies: Take letter to the Establishment Secretary.

Establishment Secretary: (Makes postings.)

The new Department

The new Station: (a) Repitition of some of the old sounds.
Patient gets in touch with old acquaintants everyday.
The new revolution in life prevails.

Presentations

Doctor Endeley and Mr. V. Tanka give presents. Patient stretching hand to receive presents for the journey.

Doctor Chinda: Going through my left toe, advises me to be firm, and to fear no body.

THE COURT - PART II

Crime and Imtimadation

Chief Justice: Once again I have come here today to hear the final findings of the last case which owing to its untraceable source, I bid you and your Secretary to investigate thoroughly before I give my final verdict. This particular case has been boiling my mind and looks strange. I am sure honourable Prime Minister, his Secretary and others concerned have been able to find out the culprits responsible for this mischief which I may term the most "treacherous crime" I have ever heard of in this country. It has come to my understanding that a soul was merely used as a political weapon.

Prime Minister: Your worship. It has not been an easy thing, it has not only touched your nerves as a lawyer but also mine and many as ordinary citizens of the state. It has not only brought sadness to the affected but it has assasinated quite a good number of innocent citizens. I, my Secretary and other colleagues have worked very hard and it is only by the sweat of our brows [128] that we were able to get a few hints on which to build our findings. As you already know such cases, like this, I have warned those responsible and have made personal interviews with those concerned. It was not only confined to the town, to the offices, to the market places and to the great amazement even to the churchs but all over the country, the nuisance multiplied by lifts and bounds.
I have been thinking of what I must suggest to you about this. We can only maintain a proper discipline and the abolition of such crimes by making a law on this into immediate effect.

Chief Justice:

That indeed has not been a small task. It has cost you and everyone of us a great deal. I am in line with your suggestion and is exactly what we have discussed with "members of the Bar." But I must say that you still have a great deal to do. You must expound this to the civil service and let this law be viewed with a very great concern. This nation

must revolve on equality and human respect of every citizen irrespective of his up-bringing and race. This rule must be maintained in every aspect of life. This is also applicable to the people, not only civil service servants.
Honourable Prime Minister, Rev. Men, ladies and gentlemen, I must say I am very very grateful for the much pains every one of us has taken to bring this matter to a close.
Thank you.

The Flight

Dominated by merry making in front of the house by Betty, Rose, Kitts and patient.
Here the Merry making is interrupted by Adhijo's [129] spiritual visit to Patient. After the visit there is the take off, patient goes alone and it is arranged that Rose will follow later.

Patient: Waving gaily and goes off.
He comes to a hotel on the road.
He takes food and drink. Offers a bottle of beer to the waitress but she turns down the offer.

Oxwald: Bridget, Rose Gana, Rev. Father Sullivan and his sister waiting to receive patient.

Father Sullivan: (Introduces me to Sister.)
I hope you will write to him when he is in London [129a]. Miss Conny Van Zanten who is in Holland will be in London with you and will teach you Dutch.

Bridget Awasum: I am doing nursing here in Oxwald and I have only a year to complete. I am so happy to be with you for these few hours. Imagine those good days at Buea in the club. There is nothing so pleasing to me than those youthful days. (At this patient and Rose Gana bid goodbye to them.)
(Rose and patient go to London. Rose Gana whose father had sent patient 10,000 francs to her agreed to put patient through his biology. He was soon introduced to his Biology and Chemistry, Teachers. Encouraged to work hard on Chemistry [130].)

END OF THE PLAY

By B. N. TANKA

PART III - COMMANDS - EVIL - MY HEALTH SINCE MARCH 19th 1968-1970

1. At 8 p.m., I sat by my table reading a book. Suddenly I heard a hideous and terrifying voice which said, "The Prime Minister has asked you to walk to the door, stand on your heels and look to the left, and right and you will see a girl whose name is Angela Ndefru by the left hand side near your window". It was a miracle, no person seen nor was there any sign that it was coming from outside. It was coming from above the ceiling. Ceiling was too weak for any weighty body to sit or stand there. The pressure pressed on me and the echoe blared poisonously into my skull. Perplexed, weak and confused, I shuffled to the door, performed the actions but being confused I did not stand on my heels. In the end I saw no one but loneliness and Moonlight.

2. With heavy eyes and head, I was in deep thoughts but being confused, I did not know myself. I sat down and in a while the voice of Mr. Andela who was then Secretary to the Prime Minister commanded me to buy some drinks, bread and magerine. As my thoughts alone give me no solution, I went to bed.

3. At about 1 a.m., I felt something pricking my back (as I lied on my back). I heard something speaking and moving in my chest. It introduced it self to be Mr. Andela. He said "we are here with Doctor Lantum". Whatever was the education, till now everything remains peculiar althought I have deduced my own conclusions. No one has been able to tell me what it was. But much foolery from people after this time everywhere in the country gave me grounds to say something. This occurence was too strange to me and I was confused and worried the more.

4. By break of day, I recognised two shadowy figures by my bed to be those of the people who were moving "in their form" through my veins and expanding them and causing me to be more thirsty than ever before. I glanced under my bed and recognised something like a snake, but as I was hurrying for Mass, I ordered my brother to check up what it was. Just when I stepped out of my house I heard the voices speaking to me right above me but I did not see anything. A severe pressure on my nervous system and weakening of my body as a whole. The chief speaker of the voices was the Secretary to the Prime Minister. His speech was full of advice and warnings. I went along the road hearing the voices.

Half the distance, a girl whom I know was speaking to me. These people were not at the time in the locality where I was. Hence it was a dead blow to my health as there was none to bring back my mind to me. I was bearing these tortures until I got to the curch. No one passed me on the way. Every place was so quiet, a condition which has never prevailed before. Until I entered the church, I was still confused and yet again a series of voices criticised me here and there and a Rev. father calmed me. Not the one who was saying Mass but one in that same spiritual form. But he was moving within me. The voices told me that there were many but as a child I could not see them. They talked of my having a family of 163 which was still strange to me.

5. After the Mass, I had to go to the market to purchase the requirements demanded by the voices.

6. I went back home instead of to the office at the command of the voices. There was something like moving in rythm with the voices.

7. I feasted in pains and was ordered by Mr. Andela to leave a loaf of bread and Magerine for the girl who was speaking to me.

8. At the end I must go to the office and the voices asked me never to go by the road through the hospital by night because of evil spirits, to go always along the road to know who would give me a lift. (A very severe shrieking voice into my ears).

9. I could not work as I was so weak in the office. I left and went home and passed to the local M. O. who gave only a few tablets to me but said that my illness was such that could not be treated in the Cameroons, as there was no Specialist.

10. I was in the parlour thinking. A fly dropped onto my left hand and walked up it and in a while. I felt some pain as it pierced through. Later there was a movement and some talking within me. It was by introduction, Dr. Lantum. He talked to me, really many things.

11. Three ghosts which I could recognise viz coming in with fright and cold air laddened with moisture.

(1) "Christine Fontam" (it might have been impersonification) came in and walked across my radio. I was petrified. Its body was quite bare.

(2) The next was ghost of "Berta" it bounced on my stomach three times.

(3) The next was in a type of skin of snake and represented "Rose" and laid down by my side but was somewhat angry, beating her legs on the bed and lastly fell under the bed and disappeared.

12. Two Butterflies landed on my bed curtain and Dr. Lantum was speaking within me. He told me it was the butterfly of Vincent Abang, with that of Rose. Rose was in love but was weak and needed shelter. There Vincent came to shelter her.

13. In the parlour, I suddenly sighted a girl coming in front of me. A voice, spoke to me, it was the spirit of Rose, and really it was in appearance. These scenes were a nuisance to me because they were causing pains and weakening me.

14. The same Rev. father before advised me to go to Mr. Andela, who was in the Regional Headquarters. I went to him but he claimed ignorance of the happening. I had to go back under a more severe tension of pains and heat.

15. Lying in bed, I saw a white Board appearing in my bedroom and the inscription "Queen Elizabeth II" appeared on it. After this, I saw the real appearance of the Queen. She wore a transparent apperel. (During this time only about three persons visited me). But there were all the time voices "speaking" EITHER within my body or on my head.

16. Very surprising, there was dead of silence all over the Vicinity right from the time I was possessed by Spirits. Then later after about three or four days, I heard nothing but a heap of Scorns.

The Phrases: Muaqua qua forty, Muaqua qua forty were used. Then there was some speeches made and the voices could be identified. It seemed that some officers were either questioning some girls or loving them.

17. I suddenly fell asleep and suddenly was awakened up by a sweet music being floated by a girl and later on she changed to singing, the voice of a white lady indeed!

18. The condition and pressure doubled when I saw frightful and recognisable faces, some dead spirits spoke my language and were performing exercises by the wall. They talked of German School days, football, and swimming with the snakes. Probably spirits invoke and transformed to deceive me that there were my relatives. They talked of backbone to be straightened on a bamboo.

It is but very neutral on this earth and inhuman for people to ill-treat a perplexed person and left confounded in this way. It is very questionable elsewhere in any court of law to leave a human being under such condition and make him an object of amusement everywhere in the country among the smallest and the greatest. "It is only somewhat an insane reaction."

19. By the window, I saw a crowd of people. Their appeances were so faint but I recognised some. A girl coming up and speaking to me and I also saw the "President" giving a present.

20. Prior to the above, the spirits in (18) dropped certain things on my body and my blood shook as those things landed on my body. They said they were examining me as many people in that town said that I was a wizard.

21. My late uncle, I saw him, he exhibited my life history right from childhood up to school age. He called out names of my friends. I heard some people talking in the camp that my grave was behind my house. I really saw some grass and I thought it was the grave that must have been made by someone.

22. A long Indian file in the Parlour. Saw many people, some lawyers reading, and some showing me different things.

23. Next, someone stepped out of my room like the president and made the following comments: That "in my occasion, I have been coming here in this house for protection and have found it a good place." My late uncle asked him a question. "Sometime you were travelling to a destination and I warned you not to go as there would be an accident." The president remembered the instance. My late uncle furtherly asked him whether he should come back to life? The president said that never in the history of revelation has it happened and that he was guarded by "Demons" Snakes.

24. Two girls landed on the two arms of two chairs. I really saw them. Their spirits indeed. It may be the poison that was in me was already working. They had white teeth, and sooner I heard a fly on my head saying, these are the Snakes of Helen and Betty. Sooner a fly landed on my left arm and the snake of Helen dis-

appeared and the fly was Helen and it walked up my arm and pierced through into my body and then speaking to me.

In the long run, it came out and was walking in between my legs and for the whole night, it was talking to me till about three a.m., when I got offended and it flew off. The second fly was that of Betty. It only went into my head and walked across my hand and off it went.

25. I heard of Telepathy, Opaque and Embalment. Some voice on my head said that I was going to be embalmed. Some of the voices talked of people being on the same line, Category. The other talked of the Prime Minister being on the highest line and linked to many other countries and persons of that Category.

26. Three other flies that went into me were: -

1. Hon. Lafon.
2. Hon. Jus who found difficulty at first and went back to fortify himself and lastly went through me. I heard of embalment.
3. Francis Shey.

My mother and father also went through me. They could speak good English within me. I was only breathing; who knows who were these? Spirits in transformation? They talked of 52 people going through me, the greatest embalment they said in the country (foolery).

27. Doctor Lantum talked of three Doctors that had gone through me: - Dr. Lantum, Chinda and Nasa. But people's reactions later told me that they were only deceiving and fooling me. (Compare Christ's temptation, forty days in the Desert.) All over the territory, many other things went into me and torn and enlarged, weakened my nerves but were not talking. The different tribes were all divided against me. "The Government probably has consent to this." They take a delight in what is adverse, agressive and against my health, relationship, my family men forced to be disunited. "The AIM."

28. Scraping movement near my Vertebral Column, and one of the Doctors said, they could determine my age. Some other painful movement around my waste and just below my hips and the end of my stomach. This area is giving me very acute pains. I recognised that it was a renal vein or artery of my reproductive Organs. Secondly the usual and the normal monthly (natural) discharge of Cement was completely stopped for so many months right up till now. There is something sucking me within from my observations.

29. After this, five demons of my mother's family introduced themselves to me. But I recognised some names because my mother used to talk of them. But how can they be here without any clue. They must have been invoked by a set of people. My father or parents will not teach me so treacherously without an introduction.

30. Whoever might have invoked these spirits or whatever the case may be, there was great concern of Magic and Spiritualism in signs. These spirits spoke to me while I was sitting down in the parlour. They talked of speed and lightening in Comparism with their movement.

31. Another Demon, very prominent among all others told me that he was constantly in touch with U.K. and America - speed like that of lightening - continuing he said he was invoked by someone and the girl he appeared to in a dream was a friend of mine.

32. They showed me my file from the office and what was therin. To be frank enough this Tipuan gave me no rest. He would shout in my ears, under my legs, by the window and during this time I was in a world of Spirits - there was no rest.

33. I saw very short images of persons in front of me like those of "Maquisedes". Some of these persons transformed themselves probably into the forms of those I knew or had known. But the Doctor would know more about these happenings especially the spirits of the dead invoked to suffer one. Or it may be there are some supernatural powers used for the same purpose. It becomes to me very surprising while women should concern themselves very much to this "a suspecting source."

34. As I said earlier, something like a fly which was invisible was always speaking to me. Even with a mirror I could not see it. I was informed that a car was going to bring two girls, with a radio which I had left in the town for repairs. Far off from the house, I could identify some people speaking like those girls and a car also glided by and came to a stop. I waited but no one came. I went back to bed with the doors ajar and all of a sudden I heard some footsteps by the kitchen and near the hedge, a load or so was thrown.

35. At night, I saw St. Jude, a patron Saint in time of difficulties. He told me he had heard my prayers and that I should continue to pray. He (he) said although he had passed out of this earth; yet he still like to come back for enjoyment. He said he was sociable when he was on earth and that they also have politics in their own world. He talked about injustice and justice the former of which is his enemy.

36. Tipuan talked about spirits trapping information from me even if I did not speak. Then some other thing told me that some books were stolen from my library and "they" knew the persons. The people around claimed to be wise only in their practice of using the snake, a "witchcraft" to know all about you even if you did not speak. It was so surprising when the neighbouring men and women took pleasure in what was against my health. They pretended to love me by speaking my tongue, and calling names of people I know. How they were taught this is very strange to me. You see, Sir, it is just as you as a Nigerian or so will be studying or working somewhere in Great Britain or any part of your country where your tribes men are not there. So if you suddenly hear people speaking your language and who cannot avail themselves to you but you always hear them from the distant and cannot make them out. Worst of all this happens only when you have been mysteriously taken ill. Definitely all these painful forces from all over the country and where else you may try to dodge are definitely going to ruin your life, transform your very self and you will look gloomy at everything. Especially when you realised many human torments arising from this from even the smallest member if the community as a whole. Whether it is a teach-

ing nobody knows because it does not serve its purpose. It destroys. Many reports were given to important Government strong points to stamp out the evil activities but in fact, it multiplied by lifts and bounds, so I begin to suspect what this must be. At least if it was something meant to teach me, I should not have been left in ignorance for a period of three years despite the Doctors recommendations. These are merely my views about the illness, how it started, the reactions of the population, my co-workers, and other people I had never met before. This will let you know whether this was a natural disease or illness, or it was an illness imposed onto me by evil, unselfish Citizens for their own goal.

37. Was it my parents? No. I deny this because they would not accept anything and would not like to suffer me so without telling me.

38. The cartoon of Heinekins: One of those voices ordered me to get a Cartoon of beer as my parents were coming that evening to see me. My parents cannot come without informing me. However, in that state alone, I sent for one. The spirit that was speaking to me termed herself to be a Reverent Sister. She spoke and advised me. She was with other two Sisters.

39. She talked of one Conny Van Zanten, a white, a girl whom I knew, that she would teach me how to swim with the snake. Prior to this, I had two dreams viz.

(a) I saw my officer at the time cutting off the neck of somebody.

(b) I saw a very large snake under my bed washing a thick blanket in a wash basin, and one of those voices told me that it was the snake of Conny.

40. I heard of people drinking, eating in the form of Spirits without my knowledge. I also heard of the clock speech.

41. Deceitfulness and jealousy predominated this unearthly Catastrophe. I heard of an helicopter being flown to collect my parents and many other vague stories. "It is love tragedy." However, imagine one's head in ill-health listening to many people. Hearing things which needed thinking and worst of all spirits in that case.

42. I heard of the spirit of Lonka A putting two people to a test. At this time something really used to pierce through my thoracic organs and I was feeling much pains and the dripping of blood or so. It was like a snake but one of the voices said it was the spirit of Lonka A. Even right up till now, I still feel the same movement. Whatever it may be you should imagine now my health since March 1968 till now. Something used to dig up my back bone and when this began, I felt drops whether of blood dripping down the walls of my body and spreading over my body. In my chest, during the snake-like movement there was a great flow of blood. I was tired, weak and helpless. I could not add 2 + 3 make 5.

At this strange sight, I was induced to drink much. But where-ever I went people who knew it laughed here and there, heaped Scorns and tortures to Worsen the conditions.

43. Formerly I talked of spirits examining me. There were really two spiritual examining actions. viz:

(a) Some of the Spirits who said they were my dead relatives examined me and said there was nothing in me. But that the people of that locality said that I was a wizard.

(b) Another examination was by some Londoneers who made the same conclusion and later on took some snapshots and told me that my image was seen all over.

44. Now I started hearing someone humming from the Gendarme Camp. Some of those Spirits would come to me and went there to exchange information. "It was so wonderful while rich men interested in me should not call me but to ill-treat me in this manner. " But who knows who were making these. I heard also that some veins were cut off from my chest to transplant into someone and that as I was young the veins would grow but that I should be very careful and avoid talking. I also heard of blood transfusion; that blood was being transfused from me in that form to a certain girl. I was told that there was a tank of blood in one of the Gendarme's house who was working in the witchcraft branch. It was so strange for me to hear of a Special Dept whose duty was connected with witchcraft. I also heard of my father sending money to father John in "witch-craft form." These are things which were strange to me. "Witchmoney for dowry." They said the Gendarme knew how to deal with this money.

45. Some friends who said had come to visit me from Britain were Bridget Awasum and Rose Gana. These came and went into my body before speaking to me. "People live in such forms in many countries," they said.

46. I was sent a pamphlet from Eye Hospital Kano, and one of those voices, that of a Doctor, Dr. Lantum told me to read the Section on "BLOOD."

47. I heard a speech made in my vernacular by someone whom I seemed to have recognised him by the voice. He merely deliberated on visits and associations. I saw many figures of different sizes. I was told that one could be made to understand any language should he transform himself into a "type of witchcraft."

48. The next morning, I dinned with my late uncle. He was speaking to me. I heard and recognised his voice but could not see him. But flashes of shadows were constantly seen moving on the floor.

49. A Doctor came in and assume the position of the speaker who sopke Vernacular. He stood in a horizontal position below the ceiling.

50. I was staying in a twin house and my neighbour was a Domestic Science Teacher and also a Co-worker. She has a boy friend who is a Soldier. As I was sitting down, I saw the shadow of the Doctor coming through the front door which was locked and that of the Soldier coming through the wall of the house. I was surprised. But is sat on the table while that of the Dr. was horizontally under the ceiling and after a while the two shadows disappeared.

51. I had a warning in the evening, my late uncle speaking loudly to me and telling me to leave the Parlour and to go to my bedroom. I hesitated but again I felt

a rapid movement pushing my feet from the floor. The voice come from beneath the floor, he asked me to leave and go somewhere because something serious would happen there.

52. In my bed, I did not sleep. I was worried. There was movement all over my bed like that of Maggots. I could not breath and was therefore suffocated. I heard a girl speaking to me and moving in the matress in that form - of maggots. The girl, Conny talked of going to Bamenda on transfer. She was a Dutch volunteer and really she was already in Bamenda. Before she went she came and greeted us in the office.

53. It was told me that this girl would teach me many things and that I would study with her in U.K. and she would teach me Dutch.

54. I left the following morning to consult a Doctor. Before my return a snake had beaten a daughter of that my neighbour and she died instantly in the hospital. The Doctor I consulted, sent me to another Dr. in the North of the country. I was often confused by those voices speaking to me. No seat was good to me because I was sitting on Maggots. But how this can be no one knows except those who are connected to this why the Maggots could not die when I sat on them but moved freely and disturbed me. Air pressure was forced into me from below and from above with the result that I was under a very great pressure but these had a severe effect on my nervous system and the body as a whole.

55. There was a type of sent off by a friend of mine who is a Medicine Student and two girls. I went alone. In fact I was speaking in jets. My veins or vocal cords were somewhat broken and I was only forcing out words which did not take their correct pronunciations. When I arrived at the U.K. I called to a place called Oxwald where I met a Rev. Father, Rose Gana, and Bridget Awasum. After a two hours stay, I went to London with Rose Gana. My subjects consisted of Biology and Chemistry.

56. As I am writing this, people not more spirits are commenting on it. Even in my office or outside it is the ordinary people that now repeat what was down by spirits, I therefore seem to believe that it was the work of their hands. Some of those men, no matter their status in life well read or not induldge into the nuisance which is only good to them but adverse to me.

57. In the North, I was given a test and after the test, some injections. These injections and tablets drove away the spirits from my body and what was very typical to me now as dreams. But people were joking over the situation, a condition which was too alarming to me, the sufferer.

58. The women talked impure, words on sex, managed to say some "Impure" phrases and scornful ones from my vernacular and were using them on me. How they got them I do not know. Probably they were connected with the Spirits.

59. I visited my father and spent some days with him and had some advice but was promised to come for native treatment later. I tried to compare and contrast the scene of events, but the place was so mute, none of such voices or phrases. It was quite different from the rest. But I dreamed all the same as a result of my ill-health.

60. A snake hid under my pillow in ambush to deal with me. Second instance to that which killed a girl but I discovered it at at 11 p.m. in the same twin house.

61. I reported to the Dr. who sent me to the North on my return and he after viewing the social and physical environments of the former Locality recommended for immediate transfer.

62. Administrative purposes delayed the transfer for up to 7 1/2 months and the nuisance and the ill-condition grew right into my bones. Everyone grew to know what had happened and that was used as a weapon to keep me aloof.

63. Of course, every unkind word pricked my heart like a dagger and many other confusing circumstances but the Doctor warned that I should not be challenged or irritated intellectually "or any other thing that will annoy me." This was never observed but whenever there was an attack or irritation I had to talk in order to warn the persons not to suffer me.

64. However in my new stations, I was surprised for the first time I arrived to hear some of those phrases from distant voices. I thought I was free but I was still going to a Hell. The same conditions prevailed and more other things were added to it. I concluded without hesitation that it was a plot set working against me. In the office, it was the same thing. I reported to a Senior Police Officer but there was no stop. Instead I used to hear people speaking to me from that office. I used to suspect some but when I went out to them they said nothing. They were learning or doing what from me?

65. I used to be beaten in bed at night and suffocated. In the church, I was not at rest. I could not say my prayers. I tried by all means to know those who were interested in me to speak to me so but I failed. But such talk from unknown personalities was a disease to my health.

66. I met the District Doctor several times and after a year I had to go to Buea. Before this, I consulted so many native Doctors and any reasonable person I saw said one thing or the other. Usually they talked of "invocation of Spirits."

67. In Buea, I was still under the influence of dreams. I reported to the District Doctor who recommended that I should see a psychiatric Doctor. The same Dr. I consulted at Kumba.

68. I was still under the same influence as elsewhere but I would like to add that it was a workable plan to my own findings because all the things that happened related to what happened to me from the onset.

69. I was taught sex in dreams. I saw many women not asleep but awake. I saw their nakedness, and their appearances in the form of shadows. But in dreams I used to see them distinctly. I saw someone lying on my bed like a snake and the Picture resembled that of the "Prime Minister" who started the nuisance in Kumba as stated in these notes. There was a girl in the middle demonstrating sex.

70. Voices used to speak in my head and I heard distinct sounds. I still feel streaming movements in the same way as before. The reactions of the people

speak. Same of aloofness even those who had known me before I left Buea. From what the people said or did I suggested they had been taught something which I did not know. Even now there is no difference in me as far as my health is concerned.

71. In the midst of the happenings, I often hear when asleep a single string of guitar played over my head. Usually I may be forced to a sudden sleep for about a second or so then I will hear the music from the string. This is later on exaggerated upon by the people who know what it means. They repeat the sound of that string from time to time and I concluded that they are referring to that sound.

72. A band too sometime played in the bedroom. But the mystery over all this is that when I get up or awakened by the sound of the music instead of seeing people, I hear noise from distant voices commenting on me.

73. I sometime find myself being carried to a river in a mad speed and in a second I find myself in bed awake. In other occasions I was swimming in some river and climbing rocky mountains and doing all types of things. If these are natural phenomena, I do not see why people should have much to say over them. They are connected only with me as an illness but how come they do know and amuse themselves over it even in the darkest hours when everyone is expected to be asleep?

74. As I said earlier, a fly or may be a devil was often on my head moving in my hair and speaking and sometime cracking jokes which were irksome to me; It said that it was making some fashion for me on my head. It probably had a silk-like substance or probiscis which it sent right down into my head and I felt the movement. It said it was making me opaque and that I was being embalmed and that the effect would be felt later. (Probiscis = probe-scissors? - Word-condensation or neologism? Or "proboscis" = trunk?)

75. In my bedroom, I used to see people riding into the house on their bicycles with flowers on the heads of the bicycles. One of the voices told me that they were devils. In another occasion, I was sitting down and suddenly saw a motor cycle rider riding into the house and found himself into the ground under the table. There he vanised.

76. I recognised three shadows coming into the house. The spirit spoke to me like the one which was on my head. Then I heard a chorus of song and I was told that they have come to see me because I was ill. They told me that they found their way through the town by snake fight. They told me that I should take out some beer for them. When they are in that form they drink in a magic way and one will not notice it. But that if they go far into the bush they can transform themselves and do things as ordinary men.

77. Another voice recalled me to my cousin who disappeared in school when he was taken ill. Searches made proved that he was missing. But the voice said he is in U.K. married to an English girl and that he is Director of Electrical Company and that he has a plane of his. It told me that he had passed home and that he would call to my place before going back. It told me that he is always friendly to Cameroonians who go to him in U.K.

78. When I was just taken ill, I saw someone carrying my grandmother in a chair. The action was fast but I recognised the shadow and reaction. At this time, she was still alife but ill (news of illness had not reached me). When I went home for my own treatment I saw her very ill and I baptised her, and she gave me her last blessing. On my return I later heard that she died.

79. The ghost of my grandmother appeared to me beating and asking for food and her face red with blood. I see faces or reflections in my eyes; sometime a whole head plunging into me from the head and after this, I feel a movement in my chest or stomach or in some of my veins.

80. (a) The figure 25,000 was written on my heart.
(b) 26 written on my left eye.
(c) The others 7.61 and 4.381 all written on my brain.

Sometime I see circles drawn on my brain. These reactions cause much discomfort to my eyes, mind and the whole body. Following the above though not all what has been happening to me, I am made "to look back" on what happens to me in a critical way. I recall irrelevant things very unnecessarily into my mind. But I should like to say if I were left alone without the interference of the people who worsened the condition by teaching me bad things in dreams or giving me unsound thoughts, gossips which embodied egotism and discrimination and other such talk which they said they were teaching me to be a "Jew and a man" I should not have had such a waxed mind. But now my mind can think of very foolish things or hate a person even without a cause merely because many people suffered me unjustly and never showed themselves to me.

This may even transform my very character but I do not know as you are here to correct all the irregularities which those people tended to force into me and deform my personality. I will also say that it has a psychological blow to me as it embodied a lot of inferiority complex. But these low attributes were imposed onto me through the evil spirits - like beating me in bed, tearing my inner flesh, performing acts which were supernatural and unclean to the body and mind and in short giving pain to my body. The ordinary citizen stepped into the same way, to intimidate me, threaten, show superiority by punishing or delaying to attend to me during which time he will speak by whispering and these will shock me and my nerves.

It also has a fatal effect on my social circles. Everyone I meet says one thing or other which he had formerly never used to say to me. And what they say exactly relates to my sufferings but I do not want people to do so or shed crocodiles tears. Such phrases, sounds or words are not good because they always carry me back to what I ought to forget.

To wipe this completely from the minds of people, the Dr. has to give a warning letter to the authority to exhibit at the proper places.

PART IV: DREAMS

Together with the three different accounts of his illness reproduced in the previous parts of this book, Mr. Tanka gave his doctor in Ibadan a collection of 38 dreams which he had recorded on request of a previous doctor interested in psychological aspects. This first group of dreams were dreamt by Mr. T. after his illness had started in 1968.

In his numerous letters beginning 1974 and discussed in Chapter 6 of this volume, Mr. T. rarely referred to dreams. Only in some lengthy reports accompanying letters written in 1976, Mr. T. mentions a number of dreams, intermingled with descriptions of his psychotic experiences. Together with the answers to a questionnaire, Mr. T. has sent another collection of 20 dreams on 9 June 1979, some of them dated between 27 May and 29 July 1976, some almost identical with those mentioned in a report from 2 August 1976. Possibly this indicates that Mr. T. has kept with himself a large body of notes from which he is sometimes copying, when writing to the author.

It seems appropriate to reproduce in this volume the two collections comprising 58 dreams to make the reader more familiar with Mr. T.'s thinking and feeling, although it was not possible to add the patient's free associations which a psychoanalytical interpretation would require.

DREAMS 1968

1. The dream of a bird kissing me and hovering over me, and counting from 1 - 600. At the same instance when I opened my eyes I heard a voice from a nearby house saying you shall live for long.

2. I dreamed another dream of paying tithe to the church.

3. I saw my father and mother, relatives and one Mrs. Cheyip [131] preparing for a send off.

4. I saw a priest lying down and reciting some prayers not understandable by me [132].

5. Inspite of ill-health, I was made to climb up to the ceiling in our Lady of Lourdes Secondary School. It was a risky attempt in which I almost lost my balance. Shoes were stored in that ceiling. Some dirty shoes were worn on my feet.

6. I saw a priest talking to some girls, I was standing behind a palm tree in my home with a girl and I asked the priest irronically that I will like to go with him to Nso to be his cook.

7. I saw the inscription: "NDONG" written on a board by the side of the wall. I then recollected that I had read a letter in the office which was written by Mr. Ndong who is a former president of Cameroon Students Union and now working in the same office in Bamenda [133].

8. The next day I dreamed of the same Mr. Ndong, how he blew air into my nostrils and my stomach was enlarged and I felt plenty of pains in my lungs and stomach when I woke up from sleep and for the whole day.

9. I felt some electric pricks in my body. A rope wound round one of my teeth and it was pulled with great vigour. My body was paining as though it was pinned with pins.

10. Rythmic movement of legs in bed (as of dancing). A higher officer in our office dressed in his work gowns and came out of the office.

11. A sudden blink of the eye and a movement in the brain, and a second's "doze off". Father Priestly grave was brought nearer to me and I noticed it opening instantly [134].

12. In the same manner as in (11) above, and a few yards away from Victoria General Hospital, I noticed a Car going on a strange road and it suddenly fell into a deep gorge and another gentleman was pursuing it for rescue. I recognised the first person.

13. The ghost of my late grandmother came to me and I found myself somewhere in her compound. Here I helped her to step over a small hill in the compound.

14. The ghost of my grandmother this time appeared in a very unusual manner. I was beaten by the ghost and it appeared that it wanted food. I noticed her face red with blood as though she was eating my head.

15. A certain man asked me to buy red Guinness for him in a chemist shop belonging to one Kwame.

16. My late grandmother came to visit me and on her departure I bought some beer for her. She drank some and hung the other two bottles on her shoulder.

17. I went to office and left Mr. Abang at home. When it was raining he came and gave me keys. Florence was working in one of the offices. I went home and on my return she had gone to Tiko and was only available in the office the next morning.

18. I dreamed of a nearby neighbour. I saw him when he was about eight years old, he had a light complexion. Suddenly his shadow developed to his normal size. He took a pot and laid it by my head. An old friend, Emmanuel, called round.

19. A dream about six with my people at home. (As soon as I opened my eyes I heard someone commenting on this in the vicinity).

I found myself being taught English in a class room by Mrs. Atabong. When I thought of one Mrs. Oben, I soon dreamed a dream in which I saw two army vehicles, one going to our office, and the other one coming directly towards me and vanished in my head.

20. Before I went to bed, I read two lines about Isaac Newton. In a dream I dreamed of seeing his tall personality with a bearded mouth in front of me.

21. Forceful breeze from a moving or flying thing to my bed and making me breathless.

22. I felt something like a snake in my belly producing undulations. It tried to force itself out of my mouth but couldn't and went out through the left side of my stomach with a piercing and painful force.

23. I saw some moving shadows (quite distinct). Some moved in front of me and some went out by the door. They represented ladies with nakedness expressed. This was not a dream.

24. In three instances as in (23) above, I saw my small cousin in the same way. Usually I often hear people say that if I want to live happily I must bring one of my sisters, or girl friends to the clerks or some Senior man before such activities will not be worked against me.

25. Severe beating while sleeping similar to those at Kumba, Bamenda. Someone coming out of a grave by the door similar to an incidence where I was shown an area for a grave being dug. In other dream I saw a grave in front of the door.

26. I saw a distinct figure of Captain Mbu and some figures representing Menka people. Then a Soldier holding a cutlass in crotching position (Probably this was a transformation).

27. After the serious beating by Spirits, I thought of Father Sullivan, then all of a sudden I saw his shadow blessing me with incense.

28. I experienced a voilent blast of noise in my abdominal organs. I found myself flying up above my bed and singing. (After this I felt plenty of pains in my stomach, chest and head). There was an up-thrust of impurities into my brain and a sudden dizziness and uneasiness in my brain.

29. Sitting at the table, I had a sudden doze as though some-one briskly pulled my head a little bit down. Then I saw a single file of girls with small native Bamenda bags in their hands. At this, I immediately saw a type of flame burning on my head. After this, I noticed two other persons jumping above by my side. (Then I thought of what a voice on my head told me in Kumba about making fashion on my head). I said the magic thread was probably burnt.

30. Some one drumming by my ear. The sharp noise penetrated forcefully into my eardrum and mind and woke me up suddenly. I heard some people speaking, recognised a man and a lady walking on their toes with their hands "handcuped".
I noticed another lady pulling a parachute-like jacket from her body. The other removed some earrings and placed them under my pillow, then held something like a cock with the neck off and blood dripping and she went off.

31. Cool air being blown into my head, and at the same time, I felt a snake-like movement under my bed. I also recollected a relative of mine who said he was ordered to arrest all women light in complexion because they have laughed at the Gods.

32. I dreamed many dreams. I decided to tie my head with a towel. When I slept again I recognised a Rev. Father curling on my head in snake, actually pressing with great force that I felt plenty of pains.

33. I recognised someone by a ring-like navel. The figure was that of Rose.

34. The figures 7. 61 were written on my brain and this reflected in my eyes. The other figures were 4. 381. In another instance in the church I saw the figure 26 written on my left eye.

36. I dreamed a dream holding a small child in my arms who was speaking very surprisingly like a grown-up.

37. I saw someone measuring my height as I was sleeping by lying near me. Someone raising up a black hat like a policeman was seen. A well dressed group of people of the Queen's body guard i. e. Queen Elizabeth II of Britain (connected to the story of my illness).

38. I saw a letter of foolscap size which read thus:-

"Illness or Preconceived Ideas."

DREAMS 1976:

39. I dreamed that I saw a bridge of planks over some water under some trees adorned by varieties of ropes and also some excrements. Again I often noticed excrements dropping into my skull.

40. (27 May 1976) When I tuned to BBC, I heard a broadcast on paperback or writer's views and heard something on "Mental imbecility". Then suddenly a bright word "SCOTCH" appeared in front of me.

41. (27 May 1976) As I lay down with eyes wide open, I noted a broom sweeping in my brain. It was a new broom.

42. (29 May 1976) I noted my uncle digging a road; then I noted a faint figure of my mother; again I noted my father-in-law cutting the leg of a chicken on a stone near his bush hut.

43. I noted myself and a procession of light candles going up to the Pope's Embassy, Yaounde.

44. In the evening period, I noted a red towel as if soaked in blood coming out of my face. A minute later, I noted partially white fingers stretched flat in my head. They were somewhat with twisted wrinkles as if affected by cold or just from ice.

45. (5 June 1976) I experienced the most extraordinary sleeping mode as if suffering from sleeping sickness. Usually when I get a book or any reading material and begin reading it, sleep used to be forced into my eyes as if there is some cold substance in my head that causes the sleep.

46. Again I used to have sleepless nights and as a result of this, I think throughout the whole night.

47. I dreamed that a layer of my head (outer) was screened up with a big knife,

not even an operating knife, removing some sort of remains. This was done while I was awake, unlike weakening me as it is often the case with the hospital.

48. (10 July 1976) I dreamed that I found myself speeding through one of German's trunk roads and my brother was carrying me on his back.

49. (18 July 1976) I dreamed that I was summoned to an assembly of the United Nations and noted someone snapping faces and gumming them together, mine was also snapped. We went round with some people and a Black man whipped my right hand as though I was trespassing. In response, I found out the cause and we pushed the black fellow and talked to him. We found the others running and planning evil on the other coloured men.

50. (29 July 1976) I dreamed that I found myself taking part in a ceremony as a university student.

51. When I went to Market to buy food, I heard a voice shouting out the word "Tetchad". Earlier, on the 5 April 1976, this lady took over the leadership of the great conservative party from Edward Heath. Again, in the recent elections which took place in Britain on 2 May 1979 Mrs. Tetchad won the election[135].

52. I dreamed again as I found myself in a school behaving once more as a school boy or student.

53. I dreamed a dream about Winstin Church Hill [136] but could not recollect what it was about.

54. I dreamed about university and gastric pains. Earlier, I had seen older students in age, in a university arguing about economics.

55. I dreamed as I saw a Whiteman carrying some ladies and later on he performed some type of exercise over a bridge with them who were carrying firewood. He later rode off for drinking.

56. I found myself in a dream in a newly built school talking to some pupils as one of the pupils too.

57. A group of Clan's men were talking to me and I saw a European in the moon as I looked up in the moon. Again at the same time I saw a graduate preaching politics and looking forward to go too to the moon.

58. I dreamed that I saw the Duke of Edinburgh with his child showing me some Cocoa tree and telling me that Cocoa is good for the skin or body.

Mr. Tanka concluded this collection of dreams, accompanying his letter of 9 June 1979 with the following remarks:

"I submitted two small volumes of written materials to you. After my return from Ibadan, I have observed the following things: That the information therein in my records and other activities concerning my thoughts and actions were been read secretly and reflected or cast back onto me again [137]. Many more dreams which resembled some I had already recorded and sent to you were infused into my mind. Hence I did not like to repeat recording them down to you."

PART V: THE MENKA. MR. TANKA'S ORIGIN AND CULTURAL BACKGROUND
(supplemented with ethnological and linguistic information by A. B.)

On the editor's request for more information, Mr. T. has provided a typewritten script of twelve pages on "The MENKA Tribe". The first two sections are based on this script with literal quotations indicated by quotation marks; the text of the other two is Mr. T.'s. Other sources used are listed in the References.

Origin

Mr. T. belongs to the MENKA tribe. The MENKA Tribe originates from an area north - east of Mamfe in the central part of former Western Cameroon, according to two maps drawn by Mr. T., of which one is reproduced (Figure 1). The tribe takes its name from the village Menka near River Tanjoh both shown on the map. Mr. T.'s relatives and tribesmen are living in many villages within an area indicated on the map.

The MENKA area belonged to Mamfe Division, later Manyu Division of former West Cameroon. After the Referendum of 1972 it became part of South Western Province of the United Republic of Cameroon.

Combining information of Mr. T.'s maps with geographical and street maps, a sketch was drawn of the central and southern part of former West Cameroon (Figure 2). On this sketch the MENKA tribe area according to Mr. T.'s map is indicated.

From the different maps consulted it reveals that the MENKA inhabit an area located roughly at 6° 00' northern latitude, 9° 40' eastern longitude. The area is circled in the north by mountains, according to Mr. T. called "Stone Circle of MENKA", possibly belonging to the Bamenda Mountains. In the south the area is partially surrounded by the rivers Emum and Tanjoh, at Oloronti joining into the River Mo which, east of the town Mamfe conflowing with the River Mbu, forms the Cross River.

"Four fifth (of the MENKA area) lies in the equatorial forest but the north-eastern part comprising the ATONG clan occupies the grassland area". The people mainly rely on food crop farming. Palm trees are grown to produce palm oil, palm wine, and raffia. Some rubber was tapped from wild trees; coffee farming is in an early state of development. Some hunting is done, especially in the northern part of the area. "The area is not reached yet by any motorable road". Medical services are not available and people depend on native drugs or medicines bought at the nearest market at Widekum or, after travelling a long distance, at Acha Tudig or Bamenda.

Figure 1

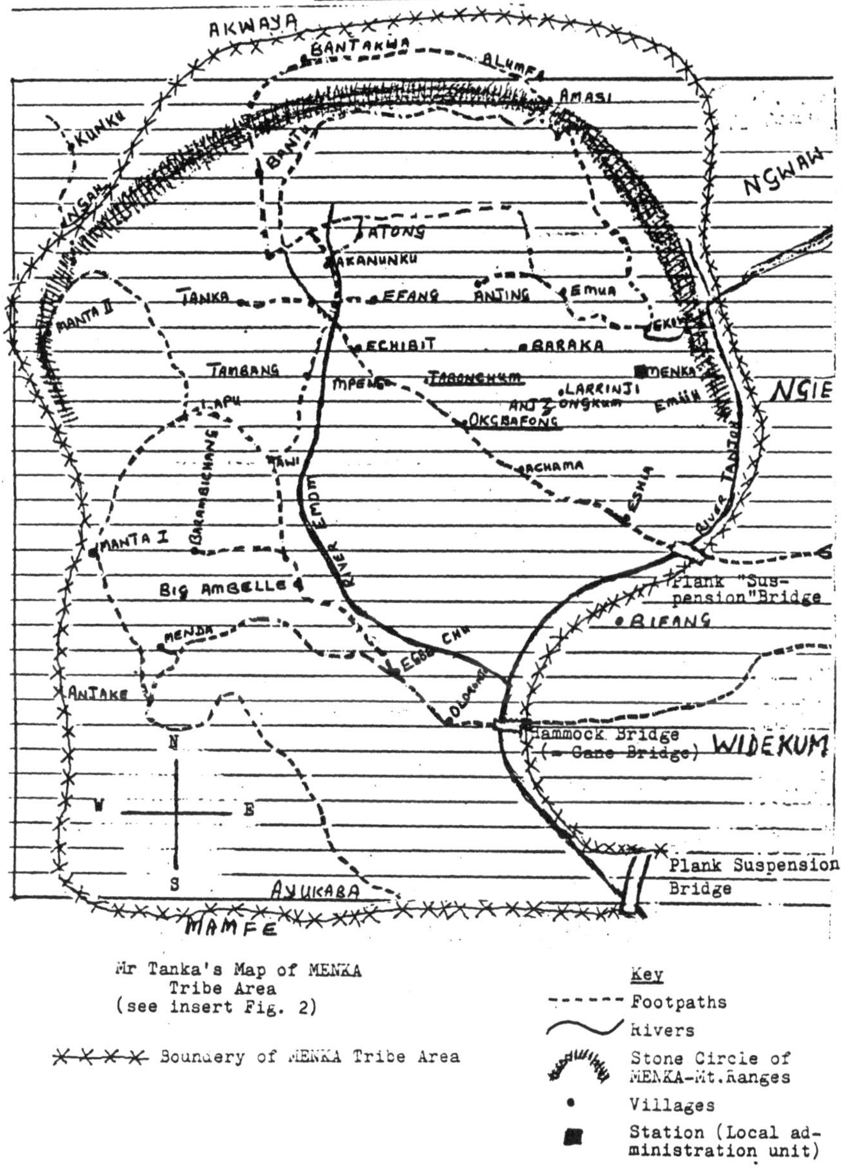

Figure 1: Mr. Tanka's Map of MENKA Tribe Area

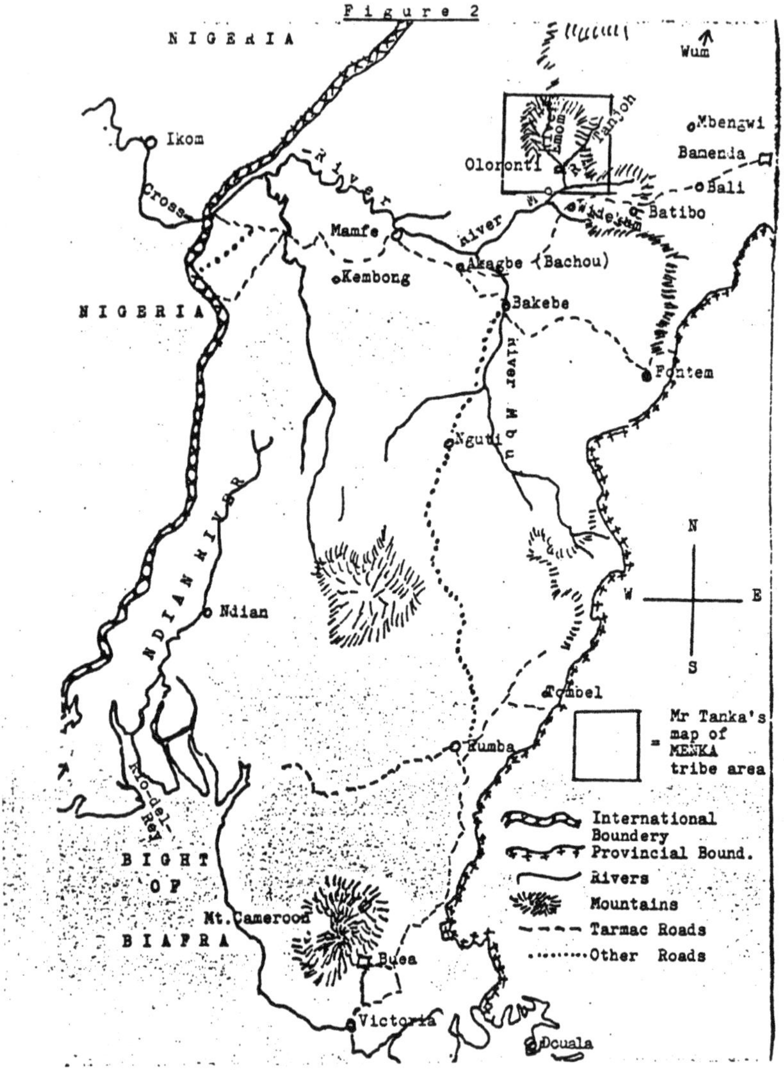

Figure 2: REPUBLIC OF CAMEROON: South Western and North Western Province (formerly West Cameroon State)

Language and Tribe

The MENKA are surrounded in the east "by the tribes of NGIE, NGWAW (NGWO), and WIDEKUM which is a twin sister to MENKA"; in the south and west by the MBO, the BANGWA, the EFANG, the MUNDANI, the BAYANGI, and the KEAKA; and in the north by the ASUMBO and AKWAYA. All these tribes mentioned by Mr. T. belonged to the same Division of Mamfe, later called Manyu.

On the map "Languages of West Africa" (Westermann and Bryan, 1952) the NGWA and WIDEKUM are noted north-east of Mamfe; the DSCHANG (= BANGWE) east of Mamfe. In the text (Westermann and Bryan, 1952) reference is made to the NGIE (p. 127) in the south-western part of Bamenda Province; to the EFANG, ASSUMBO, and KEAKA (p. 114), all three related to the EKOI dialect cluster of the TIV, spoken in southern Nigeria and in Cameroon; to the BANGWA (= DSCHANG) in the extreme east of Mamfe Division (p. 128/129); to the MBO (p. 128) living west of the DSCHANG, south-west of Mamfe. The MBO are also mentioned by Talbot and Mulhall (1962). Westermann and Bryan (1952) finally treat in some length the WIDEKUM (p. 126-128), a group of related languages, spoken "at and around Widekum between Bamenda and Mamfe" and adjacent areas of Bamenda Province. NGIE and NGWAW are thought to be related to WIDEKUM.

The suggestion the MENKA might be a sub-tribe or clan of the KOM, a subgroup of the TIKAR (Marum, 1975), is rejected by Mr. T. "The TIKARI group includes all the regions of the northern part of Cameroon... The only relationship (between the TIKARI and the MENKA) is that they are all Cameroonians". The most western of the TIKARI tribes, the KOM and FUNGOM (Westermann and Bryan, 1952, p. 123) are living near the town Bamenda which "is 62 miles or 100 km away" from the MENKA area (Tanka).

In the description of his experiences (Part II and III) Mr. T. mentions one "Honourable Lafon". Fon is the word for Chief in the TIKARI language (Marum, 1975). Mr. T. confirms that the word Lafon comes from the BANSAW (NSO) of the TIKARI tribes (Westermann and Bryan, 1952, p. 123), but "has a meaning with the TIKAR people only".

According to Mr. T. the MENKA "fall under the BANTU group which extends right to the coastal region". In Greenberg's (1955) classification of African languages the BANTU languages belong to the Central Branch of the Niger-Congo linguistic family. Besides BANTU with its hundreds of languages belonging predominantly to central and southern Africa, south of the so-called BANTU line, the Central Branch comprises 21 language groups from an area stretching from the drainage of the Cross and Benue rivers in southern Nigeria and in Cameroon to central Nigeria. These non-BANTU language groups of the Central Branch are also named SEMI- or PROTO-BANTU. The BANTU line (Seligman, 1961), starting in the west from the sea coast at the mouth of the Rio del Rey (separating Nigeria from Cameroon), runs north-east along the boundary, winding southeast with many irregularities through the Mamfe - Bamenda region, close to the MENKA area.

Westermann and Bryan (1952), however, consider this classification as premature and not yet sufficiently supported by linguistic facts. They designate all languages of central and eastern Nigeria and of Cameroon, as far as they do not belong to any of the well defined larger units, simply as "Isolated Language Group". They divide this group according to linguistic principles in "Class Languages" and "Non-Class Languages".

Although MENKA is not mentioned, it can be assumed to belong to the "Class Languages", as all languages marked on the map, and mentioned in the text by Westermann and Bryan (1952), appertaining to the area between Mamfe and Bamenda, as well as all tribes, mentioned by Mr. T. as neighbours to the MENKA, do belong to the "Class Languages".

Westermann and Bryan (1952) state further, that the WIDEKUM - "twin sister to MENKA" (Tanka) - vocabulary shows some correspondence with BANTU. Mr. T. states the WIDEKUM are similar to the MENKA in "administrative ... and tribal customs".

Considering the information available, it seems likely that the MENKA belong either to the not very well known Western Division of the Western BANTU (Seligmann, 1961), or to the related SEMI-BANTU languages of the Central Group of the Niger-Congo Family (Greenberg, 1955), probably the Cross River sub-group. In either case, the MENKA belong to an linguistically mixed area with "extreme fragmentation and intermingling of the tribes, tribal sections, 'clans', and village groups (with) every village (having) its own language or dialect often incomprehensible even in the neighbouring villages" (Westermann and Bryan, 1952).

Despite the remarkable differences in languages, the people of the region do not differ much in physique from each other, whereas there are differences in some physical characteristics compairing them with tribal groups living further west, as e.g. the IBO or YORUBA (Talbot and Mulhall, 1962).

Notes on the History of Cameroon and the MENKA Area

(written entirely by Mr. Tanka, with minor editorial changes and additions in brackets)

The coastal region of Cameroon was first explored by the Portguese in the 15th century and later by the Dutch, British and French in the 16th century. The first settlers were the British in the 19th century. After the Berlin conference of 1884, the British had to leave the country. The Germans then occupied the country and built their first office at Buea because of the favourable climate. The colonisation of the hinterland was not an easy task. Finally the land Mamfe was reached and an administrative Headquarter was created.

The MENKA people originated from Emiih and were ruled by the Chief Dikagmoh. The traditional administrative unit was at Evun Gurun in Emiih and was governed by the elders of every house or family. The members of this high council were often summoned to this assembly, to discuss the affairs of the society and individual problems.

At one time, a woman, nick-named Aquongnitichini, hanged herself after she was provoked by people who trespassed and cultivated her estate. According to the custom of the early people then, no one was allowed to live in a land where someone had commited suicide. It is further believed that crops were destroyed by wild pigs, elephants, and other plagues. Consequently, the people emigrated to Okgbafong. The administrative unit was also transferred to this new environment. There was constant fighting amongst the citizens at Okgbafong resettlement area until the first world war broke out. The effects of this caused some of the people to emigrate to Ambelle and the rest to Tabonchum. Here the centre of the local administrative unit was located at Evuntab at Tabonchum. In the same manner as at Emiih and Okgbafong, it was ruled by the elders of the society who were elected from every house and family.

A German Whiteman called Tabong (perhaps a wrong pronunciation of a foreign name) set the town on fire. This let the people to emigrate to Anjzongkum, where they stayed for about a year. Then they were attacked by a plague of jiggers which killed many men and women. This caused the people to emigrate to the villages of the MENKA clan and to those of the ATONG Clan which then was ruled by Chief Mberabah.

Although the MENKA Clan and the ATONG Clan were separated by strife and misery, yet they had a common local judicial link where the problems of the society were settled as well as important ceremonies.

After the first world war the English occupied one sector of the country and the French the other one. The administrative units created by the Germans were maintained by the English in what was then known as British Cameroons. The District Station at Mamfe continued to administer the tribes of MENKA, WIDEKUM, AKWAYA and the rest of Mamfe which included KEAKE, MBO, BANGWA, MUNDANI, BAYANGI extending to Manyemen. Only the NGIE and NGWAW tribes were shifted northwards into the Bamenda Province.

The Native Administrative Unit was under the leadership of a Court Clark and was represented by a chief from each village. A president was elected from among the chiefs and his word was final and respected in any judgement.

(In the script of Mr. T. follows a passage describing intertribal wars and the taking of slaves, including fighting episodes with "enemy soldiers". These events are attributed to the second world war although they seem more likely to belong to the first world war. The passage is left out.)

Cameroon obtained Independence on January 1st, 1960. In a plebiscite of 11th February, 1961 the Southern British Cameroons decided to join the Cameroun Republic, which then, on 1st October 1961, became the Federal Republic of Cameroon. The former British Southern Cameroons was named West Cameroon and became a sovereign state within the Federation, with her capital at Buea.

The administration of West Cameroon carried out some political changes. Thus, the MENKA tribe, formerly under Mamfe Division was placed under the newly created Division of Gwofon. Plans were continued by the new Prime Minister, Solomon Tandeng Muna, who took office in January, 1968. (Solomon Tabeng Muna, born 1912, belongs to the META = MENEMO tribe, of the WIDEKUM language group according to Westermann and Bryan, 1952, p. 127, living north-north-west of Bali, very close to the MENKA area, in the Bamenda District. He is the son of a fortune teller. Schooling in Bamenda. 1932 teacher in Bali, then Teacher Training College in Kumba. 1947 Tutor at Batibo. 1949 London. Since 1951 active in politics. Several terms of office as Minister. Segal, 1961).

The new Division of Gwofon was later removed to Mbengwi. These changes influenced the way of life of many people and created quite some problems especially in the administration.

Five years after the reforms of 1967 in West Cameroon, plans for having a unitary state instead of federalism were started. The plans were to be implemented on the basis of a Referendum which took place on 20th May, 1972. At this Referendum the majority opted for a unitary state. Very soon afterwards the French way of administration was introduced. Yaounde became the central administrative unit and capital for the United Republic of Cameroon. Everyone experienced problems arising from the new ways of administration, especially within the hospital and school services. Many loop-holes are created in the entire machinery of government in every service everywhere.

Religious Beliefs, Rites and Customs of the MENKA
(written also by Mr. Tanka)

The MENKA people always believed in the existence of God and observed their customs very strictly as the least disobedience might provoke a curse from God on the individual concerned. All ceremonial activities were first consecreted to God before the people joined in to eat or to dance. Special rites were performed to God before the beginning of every farming season. Also the first fruits were offered to God at every harvest season. Special rites were observed after the birth of a baby and also at the death of any class of persons.

The customs or traditions of the MENKA people in all three clans are the same, with the exception of the AMBELLE clan; they have the Anyangkwa society, a special society, which is a borrowed custom from the BANYANGI tribe (possibly related to the BALI according to Westermann and Bryan, 1952, p. 122). The tradition includes various societies. Each society is governed by rules or laws. Admission into each society can only be done by fulfillment of conditions laid down by the Ancestors. However, in some of the clans some of these conditions have been altered.

The Enjiti or Juju society is, from time eternity, strictly patronised or enjoyed by men who have joined it after fulfilling the conditions. No woman is allowed in this society, no matter what her qualifications may be or how much money is being paid. Even food or wine drunk or eaten in this society cannot be given to a woman. No admittance of any person or sex in any form, concrete or supernatural, is allowed in this society.

The Enkuczhong society is also a society for men only and strictly forbidden for women. Only men who are qualified by fulfilling the conditions are allowed to join the society. Drinking and eating though is enjoyed by both men and women, as well as children. Women have their own share of food and wine outside but join in the merry making.

The Ankiafong society is a women's society. It takes place seldom, only once in a while when because of a very big crime it is deemed necessary by the women. It is intended for grown-ups. The person inviting this society to her aid and support must pay the members in money or in kind. Its activities consist of dancing and singing around or through the affected vicinity, usually at night and in stark nakedness. Any man or boy found trespassing will be punished accordingly.

The Enchubuh society is ruled by the men who have got entrance into it by fulfilling certain conditions. Among them, few people are selected whose duties are to take the lead in the dance, and to kill the animal for the dance. No woman is admitted to the house, but many other people including women may participate in the dance, in certain actions, and in drinking and eating. Many other names are given to this type of society, as Wutatulu, Epam, and Wakan. They differ only by slight varieties of the dancing steps.

The Awuyom and Tangwotah dances are women's dances usually on ceremonial occasions or for entertainment. Men and children do also participate. It is free to join the dance, but the woman who invites for the dance usually feeds the attendents very well. If the dance is for entertainment, there may be little or no eating and drinking.

The Anduroh and Denkuh dances are dominated mostly by women, but men and children may take part as well. They are usually performed for ceremonial occasions as well as for entertainment. In either case food and drinks are essential.

Death Celebrations for men and women, who have attained the required age, are determined by the elders of each house. Dates are fixed for the celebrations. People look forward to have a worded account of this to avoid cheating. Death celebrations cost a lot of money and worries. The Juju dance is usually performed at the death ceremony of a man, and the women's dance at that of a woman. With the exception of the Juju dance other classes of dances or societies can be celebrated in the case of a woman or even a man, which also applies to young men and women.

Birth Celebrations take place after the circumcision is performed. The hair of the child is shaved and is usually preserved, together with the cord under a plantain stem. Food and drinks are passed round for drinking and merry making. It is a sort of prayer and welcome address to the new born baby as well as a relieving factor to the mother for the pains she bore when the child was in the womb and at delivery. When the plantain later bear fruits, they will be eaten officially by the parents and near relatives of the child.

These rites and ceremonies are difficult for indigenous citizens to carry them out outside their homes owing to lack of the necessary means because of high prices of everything.

Certain rites are performed at Planting and Harvest Seasons. There is a special place, located usually under a big tree which is cleaned and weeded for the ceremonial rite. Food, wine, a fowl or an egg are the ingredients for the sacrifice. The fowl is killed and blood sprinkled either on the ground or into an already dug pit. Wine is also poured into the pit. At the different stages, the chief celebrant says prayers to God for a good yield, asking Him for good crops. The fowl is then roasted on a fire and shared amongst those present. If an egg is used instead of a fowl, prayers are said, the ceremonial ground and the people are blessed, and then the egg is flung very far away.

Various customs regulate Marriage and Sex Relations. In the old times a girl was allowed to attain full maturity before she was given for marriage. As time went by, young men wanting to settle down early used to go in for marriage with girls of only sixteen years old and little above. The normal age of marriage for the boy is now about 20 years. Those attending post-primary eduaction often reach 25 years and above before being able to marry.

Sex is not allowed until a lawful marriage is established. Any illicit sex with a girl or a married woman is punishable by native laws and customs. A very heavy punishment is imposed by native sanctions and sometimes also by the Court. Parents often guide their children from the clutches of untamed people, whom I may call 'wolves in sheep's clothing' or 'unrespectable gentlemen'. Sex being complicated should never be tested outside of marriage.

By Christians sex is only enjoyed in marriage. The word 'sex' sounds very sweet and enjoyable to any mature girl or boy and even to a man or a woman. Just as it sounds 'sweet', it also sounds delicate and complicated, particularly to poor children from poor families or tribes who are novices. Even experienced children should not attempt it. Novices and also experienced children both have their own penalties. Most of the deaths and fatal diseases are contributed by illegal sex.

Adultery and fornication are forbidden and punishable by the churchs (by repentance, confession and forgiveness), by tribal laws, and by the penal code. By tribal laws, offenders may be cursed with snake bites, accidents, and many other misfortunes. In addition, a fine may be imposed.

Tribal investigations are taking place in cases of suspected illicit sex. The female suspect is usually cross-examined by the parents. When unwilling to admit the accusation, she will be forced to swear or take an oath. In this case, some native medicines are used. If the suspicion was wrong, the suspect will not be attacked by any illness on swearing the oath; but if the accusation is genuine, she will fall sick. She will then be asked to name the illicit sex doer.

The culprit will then be penalised, either traditionally or by penal code, whereas the girl will then be given some medicine to recover from the illness. The male culprit is cross-examined in a similar way and fined or punished.

Rape is a very big offence and is strongly forbidden. Offenders are heavily punished by native laws and by penal code.

Conversations on sex or sexual actions should never take place in the presence of little children as they are very witty to imitate our actions or habits. God himself has warned us that a stone will be tied to the neck of anyone, and he will be thrown into the deep, who deceives the little ones, for such is the kingdom of heaven. - Sex should only be taught to children who are soon reaching maturity. All teachings should be based on warnings and advice. Mature girls often want to experiment what they have been taught and thereby go the wrong way, and become stubborn to society and everyone else. Sex is a barrier and a weapon to progress.

The Christian marriage is usually monogamous. It can only be contracted among Christians, and usually within the third degree of kindred. According to the customs of the MENKA people, it can be contracted within the fourth or fifth generations. This law is strictly observed. In some families marriage may take place only from the fifth generation upwards. Polygamous marriages with more than one wife are very common among non-Christians. Intertribal marriages have often been a failure, as from time eternity the customs of the MENKA people have been adhered to strictly which seems very strange for foreign wives to observe.

Family life of the MENKA follows the common rule that the father is the head of the family and the mother is the keeper of the house. The mother and the children are depending on the father whose decisions have a final say in family problems. It does not mean that whatever the father says is correct. Sometimes, he can be guided by the wife, and then he will say something reasonable and profitable to the family. Hence, the government of the family lies in the hands of the father and husband.

Close relationships between the extended family is a natural phenomenon in every family in Cameroon, Africa, and even Europe. The people of MENKA trace the family tree or relationship very far up to the last limit if possible. We, the MENKA people, believe in brotherhood, sisterhood, cousins, nieces, aunts, uncles, and nephews as well as relations of other wives of the same father or the same parents. This is a stronghold for the government of the family, which creates good moral conduct, discipline, responsibility, and respect for human beings. Hence, a combination of various families constitute a nation. Disciplined and responsible families will make a good nation, where will reign equality, peace, justice and respect amongst all the citizen.

When one is highly committed morally, there will be no evil in his mind towards any person; but a lonely man thinks only of himself and his heart is always thinking of evil plans and achievements. In this respect, I will recommend to the Government of this country to encourage family life rather than scathing or wrecking families or homes for the sake of "Politics" which are enjoyed by only a few.

Common diseases are treated locally by herbalists. Some patients are using whiteman's drugs to cure themselves. Very severe cases are taken to the hospital for treatment. This is a very big task as communication by any means is difficult. To carry a patient on the back or on a locally made stretcher for very long distances is a burden both to the patient and the carriers.

It is a common belief that Witchcraft does exist in every society. Witchcraft is somewhat like a gift to some families which others have not. In early days the activities of witches or wizards were very common in every society. As they used these means to destroy lives or to cause damages to properties of others they died. When good citizens saw that these activities were destructive to lives, to morale, and to progress, they decided to control witchery action.

In the villages of the MENKA tribe the native doctors or medicine men passed a law not to treat anyone who was found preying on other men's life or blood. The only alternative for this evil doer was death. This action caused many deaths. As a consequence, witches and wizards had to be on their look out.

Witchery hunting is strictly limited within the domain of the village. No one can cross the boundery of the village land. In the tribal witchery hunt the law remains the same. By the custom of the tribe witchery fighting or enmity is only common amongst the citizens of the village or of the tribe, i.e. the indigenous citizens. Hence no MENKA man can hunt by witchcraft beyond the limits of his tribe. Witchery hunting for wealth is punishable by death. Witchery hunting in the MENKA is done nowadays only for the killing of animals in the forest. In some tribes in Cameroon or in Africa, people have no control over their natural gifts like witchcraft and tend to cause trouble with everyone they meet. God actually had a purpose when he created these gifts. They were meant for the protection from harm of the enemy, or for pleasure, or for help to escape from attack, but not for humiliation, or for demoralisation of character, or for isolation.

The first Christian denomination introduced by the missionaries was the Roman Catholic Faith. It is a common belief that too many forms of faith will confuse people trying to understand God. There should be only one faith until the citizens are ripe enough to understand themselves and to choose between right and wrong. However, the north-eastern part (of the MENKA area) is predominantly Presbytarian.

5. ANNOTATIONS TO 4.

PART I:

1. "He was my schoolmate in a senior year and he tried to help me for two years. I have met him again several times. He and Dr. Lantum were from the same school."
2. An acquaintance; her father put the patient in charge of church meetings.
3. "She is really called Rosita, my first girl friend. The name "Lonka A" is a nickname taken from a name of some sweets."
4. "Gabriel Tanke" - he is a classmate of the patient.
5. "This is not true, but an invention, poetic liberty."
6. In this paragraph there are religious connotations, some platitudes, some mystical meanings.
7. Neologism?
8. People in the shape of flies were sitting on his head, advising him and talking to him.
9. Christine and Betty are two different people.
10. When seeing this specific shadow he always started laughing.
11. A phrase without meaning to the patient.
12. Ideas of influence
13. Écho des pensées
14. Patient explained his spelling of "flute" as float, that the music produced was "floating around". So the spelling was intentional and can be interpreted as neologism or condensation of thought.
15. Contradictory words used together ("music blared so sweet").
16. Names of deceased people.
17. Écho des pensées. In the following "film strip thinking".
18. "Concentration camp" means: army camp. The patient explained "I call it concentration camp to express that everything is concentrated there because most of what has happened to me was coming to me from there" - over conclusive thinking. The following "Over sasse order" is in pidgin English and means "things which have been long waited for" - according to patient's explanation.
19. This is almost like poetry; it could remind one of Walter von der Vogelweide.
20. Patient's spelling - he meant uttered.
21. "The snake girls in love with each other" was explained by patient as "a symbol of love"; the implication did not become quite clear.
22. Tactile hallucinations.
23. Simultaneousness of experiences.
24. Feeling of bodily change.
25. The spelling and meaning was discussed with patient. Apparently he meant "semen" but stuck to his original spelling. This might be explained by overconclusive thinking (semen when drying in sticky - and so is cement..).
26. Revolutionaries in the bush.
27. A special type of witchcraft by which humans transform into snakes. In the following the patient is referring to thought reading.

28. Patient felt as an "experimental tool" to some scientists, confirming that quite clearly during discussion.
29. Refers to pictures in an issue of the Old Testament he has seen.
30. St. Jude is a saint the patient used to pray to; he is responsible for difficulties. Alliteration?
31. Father John is the priest of the locality. The comment "slept with me in the bed in his spirit" has no further implications according to patient's explanation.
32. Patient explained: "Without saying anything they could get my thoughts." The word "trap" might be a contraction of trap (to catch in a trap) and tap (to tap something from a well). Thought withdrawal.
33. An example of the use of stereotypes.
33a. This is an unusual spelling of "Carton of Heineken (beer bottles)". Neologisms? Mistakes?
34. "Shooting out a long tooth from his mouth"? Mr. Elonge is the patient's boss.
35. Bizarre expression: altering the usual "cold" war into "cool" war. He explained that he has used the expression "cool war" because it was done in a mystical way, the only sufferer being himself.
36. Conny is a Dutch girl teaching at a school.
37. Déja-vu.
38. First sign of insight?
39. This story of the snake the patient could not understand. He thought even if the Uncle was a wizard, it is not clear how the snake could survive. No further explanation obtainable.
40. Patient did not correct this formulation of the proverb when going through the typed test. Only when he was referred to it he realised that his formulation was not correct. - Schizophrenic distortion of a proverb is likely.
41. Contraction of "relief" and "leave".
42. Memories of his school lessons or his reading and, at the same time, alliteration to "lance"; one could call it a "schizophrenic pun".
43. People were talking behind his back; they were making teasing derogatory remarks. This is elaborated in the whole paragraph.
44. Ambivalent feelings towards his experiences; being in grief with pain and also being amused by the remarks of the people.
45. Feeling of special importance; almost grandiose ideas.
46. Insight increases. Patient is consulting the traditional healer. He also continued his treatment with the medical doctor very conscienscíously as he reported.
47. Depersonalisation. He was the "National Character", in a way replacing everyone.
48. Thought reading. Patient explains: "Thoughts which were not in me were forced into my mind."
49. "Telepathy" means that his mind was read by another person.
50. In the same paragraph reference to thought reading and influencing of thoughts.
51. There are some distorted proverbs in the last two paragraphs.
52. This paragraph is a summary of Part I; it is an illustration to pseudophilosophy and mystical thinking (Mayer-Gross, page 267).

Part II:

53. Distortion of the word "calamities".
54. Contraction of "probe" and "project" and of "breath" and "breadth".
55. Connections are not understandable or logical on first glance. Patient explained that "He (the Prime Minister) had been a Prince already for three months which he realised only afterwards." The explanation follows in the next paragraph and indicates clearly "symbolism".
56. Patient used to read "The Plain Truth" for many years and stopped only in 1969. The book seems to be a popular treatise.
57. Patient explains: "The other one is really Rose. Everything concerns him and the girl." Rose is a girl he met in 1967. He became friendly with her. He proposed marriage to her, but she could not give any reply before she finished school. She is now teaching (1970). The spelling "heroe" and "heroeine" is old-fashioned; a mannerism.
58. Patient uses this word with the meaning of "dirty"; pressed for further explanation he states: "The use of slang, using conventional expressions in an ironical mode; using foul language in a hidden way."
59. The designation of the play as "Tragedy" and "Comedy" could indicate some ambivalence. Patient explains the play is transforming into a comedy "because it ends in triumph".
60. Patient explains: "Whenever I was alone I was hearing voices commenting on my thoughts. If two friendly people are together speaking their minds, nothing could remain to be read."
61. This rather pompous expression has a strange double quality. In one way it is quite serious used in a naive way; but at the same time it sounds like the ironical way of a jester. This impression is enforced when talking it over with the patient and by the patient's explanation: "It refers to my illness. One of the flies (alliteration) said I could go to England to do medicine."
62. A Swiss doctor working at a Mission Hospital in Acha Tugi.
63. "Kits is somebody's name, abbreviated for Christopher."
64. "Rose is just everything good combined."
65. This is, of course, the patient depicting himself.
66. "The snakes fought with their knees..." - remains obscure.
67. In the description of the characters he uses a lot of cliches; Handworking" (instead of hard working) appears repeatedly and seems to be a neologism rather than a spelling mistake. E.O. = Education Officer.
68. According to patient "Well known politician."
69. A Dutch girl he has met.
70. "A friend who took me to a native doctor."
71. Patient puts together at least unrelated, almost contradictorary characteristics.
72. "To visit the patient in the hospital."
73. "If you love a person very much without return; you suffer from love sickness and become careless; your socks may slip."
74. Spelling of the patient!
74a. "To ample" = archaic for "To amplify".
75. "This is a metaphor."
76. Stereotyped expressions.
77. "What you have been hiding from a person: speak it out. Bladder is used as a metaphor for mouth." Bizarre expression.

78. This refers to a previous line: "Love knows no pleasure in miniature" (the fourth verse of this poem).
79. Patient explains: "I have been sick for two years and you have not come to see me." (Meaning the person addressed in the poem).
80. "Somebody treated like a slave, who has to play his part only in the kitchen."
81. "On earth we differ; when we die we all sit on the righthand side of God."
81a. "Amoungst" could be a contraction of "amongst" and "amount".
82. Neologism: apparently a distortion of "co-operation" but keeping some of the meaning of "corporation" as well.
83. Porcupine (expression in pidgin english).
84. The whole poem but especially the second half is a strange mixture of banalities, wisdom and even poetic beauty; in a part, as the patient states, it is "like a prayer."
85. Patient's explanation: "Many students graduate at one time."
86. Patient explains: "When I was ill I had to do something to keep my mind busy; therefore I wrote the play - when I came to this place I was still suffered by the same people."
87. Distorted word; it is meant "uttered".
88. Spelling mistake or distortion.
89. There is some insight dawning on the patient when he is writing this part. Patient elaborates on his earlier experiences: "Everything and everytime the voices were talking, advising etc." The patient reports that the voices would repeat what he wrote down when making a shopping list. He did not like this experience and he was losing his health.
90. The ambivalence of patient's attitude towards his experiences is well described in the play by the different characters.
91. Tactile hallucinations.
92. Écho de pensée.
93. Patient did smell the odour: olfactory hallucinations.
94. See note 11; no meaning.
95. See note 14; in regard of the spelling of "float", instead of the correct "flute".
96. The likening of death with (mental) illness is quite pathetic.
97. Thoughts being put into his mind.
98. Patient states: "Where I come from there are only two secondary schools, Sasse and Bale." No further explanation given.
99. No translation obtained. Patient reports that words were forced on his mind only on the first day. Patient explains further: "Only later ordinary people like uneducated women were talking about sex which might be clean to them but dirty to another person." No further clarification obtainable.
100. See note 30. This might be an alliteration: "The Jew is St. Jude".
101. This and other words and expressions indicate the strong influence of the Mission School on patient's language.
102. "Écho d'action."
103. Patient explains: "They were using some words in my native tongue which were not good and were relating to sex. It might have been bad to my mind. These words are not necessarily dirty in my language."

104. "I became afraid of myself. Nothing in my mind was my own. They were reading my mind. I became very suspicious of myself. My thoughts were not mine but were studied by some other people. "
105. Déja-vu (?)
106. Patient belongs to the numerous group of people who are working and studying in the evening for educational qualifications.
107. A good sample of the matter-of-fact way in which patients are combining Western and traditional treatment, especially, of course, in cases like this one. It also indicates a fair amount of insight into his being ill.
108. According to the medical report by Dr. Schwarz a Rorschach Test was administered which was "not very pathological". (See Dr. S.'s report.)
109. Patient apparently resented psycho-dynamic interpretations given by the doctor interested in psycho-therapy (?).
110. Patient adds: The medicine will improve his complaints in different organs: skull, stomach, liver, chest. The later development of his condition with somatic projections (hypochondrical complaints) coming more and more in the foreground is here preformed already.
111. This is very suggestive for psycho-dynamic interpretations.
112. Letter by Dr. D. N. Lantum of 17 June 1968.
113. Typical interpretation of traditional healers to put the blame on another person, thereby encouraging paranoid ideation.
114. Describing some of the methods of traditional healers by the patient.
115. The patient is weighing the advantage of the traditional healer against the western-trained doctor in a matter of fact way, not differing much from a patient in other parts of the world who considers which hospital he should consult. There is no perception recognisable of a basic difference between the two.
116. Once and again flashes of insight are recognisable, which were not present in Part I. "S. S. P." equals abbreviation for some of the officers in his department.
117. The two girls are Florence and Bridget whom he knew before.
118. These thoughts are put into his mind; they include neologisms.
119. Once again it is remarkable how well the patient relates the attempts of explanatory psycho-therapy of his previous doctor.
120. This illustrates the attitude of an experienced western-trained doctor; if a patient expresses the desire to see a traditional healer he will not oppose this wish.
121. The traditional healer also appreciates the western medical methods....
122. This is the name of the traditional healer's place; there is no special meaning discernable; although there is some reference to London, U.K., at the end of the play. Loose associations?
123. It is thought by some authors that the need for an interpreter for a psychiatrist from abroad may impede his usefulness with his patients of another language. In the case of a traditional healer, this does not seem to matter.

124. "To make love" is not used with a sexual meaning.

125. Patient describes medicine as very powerful. He was in bed for the whole day. His eyes were turning all the time. He could not "Say anything correctly" before the effect of drugs passed. This looks much like the effect of Rauwolfia (Prince,1960).

126. Cuts were made on the back, both hands, on the chest, one on the right leg and the one in the neck. Further descriptions of the traditional healer's activities, which could be differentiated as magical (cuts), encouragement or acting out (slapping the stone), autosuggestive (repeating sentences) and again magical (dropping sticks into a river which will take them away along with the illness (Prince & Speed, 1963).

127. This is a bit mixed up. Patient apparently is now reporting again to a Government doctor.

128. Once again stereotyped expressions.

129. The President of the Cameroons.

129a. This is the name of the traditional healer's place; there is no special meaning discernable; although there is some reference to London, U.K., at the end of the play. Loose associations?

130. The meaning of the last few paragraphs is not quite clear. Patient explains: "One of those flies (sitting on his head) told me that a certain man would give me money to be taught these subjects. The girl would introduce me."

Part IV:

131. Dream 3: Mrs. Cheyip is the mother of Rose who figures prominently in Part I and Part II.

132. Dream 4: The priest was lying down flat on his stomach.

133. Dream 7: "Ndong" is a name of an officer in the Civil Service whom the patient knows.

134. Dream 11: Father Priestley was an English priest who taught at a college. The patient only knew his grave since the priest had died before his time.

135. Dream 51: Misspelling of the name of Mrs. Thatcher may have a special meaning not recognizable from the material available.

136. Dream 53: Notice the spelling of Winston Churchill's name, which also implicates a special meaning but is easier to recognize.

137. Concluding remarks: Examples of thought reading and of thoughts being forced upon his mind.

6. PSYCHIATRIC COMMENTS

6.1 Editorial Aspects

Seven years have passed since, in 1973, Mr. T.'s manuscripts were transscribed, annotated, and prepared for publication.

Much more material has become available. Up till now, when the final manuscript of the book is being written in 1979/1980, Mr. T. has sent to the editor 43 letters consisting of about 150 densely written pages. The letters and attached scripts, differing in length, style and content, include additional accounts of his experiences, one of 21, another one of 20 pages, some more dreams added to Chapter 4, Part IV, an essay on Mr. T.'s tribal background, presented as Chapter 4, Part V (with minor editorial changes and somewhat supplemented), and replies to three questionnaires (1974 and 1979), which together with excerpts from the letters constitute the basis for the Follow-up 1974 - 1980.

It was tempting to include all additional writings of Mr. T. in this volume. Practical reasons spoke against it. The patience of the reader will be tested already by the triple narrative of Mr. T.'s experiences, as a plain story, a play and a summary. To add more versions would have been too much. Readers of the preliminary draft recommended shortening or omitting parts of the original manuscript. This advice, though, was not followed, as the three parts constitute variations of the same theme, resulting in some thing which has a certain literary and artistic quality. Studying the work in toto gives the reader a unique opportunity to become familiar with the working of this "African Mind in Health and Disease" (Carothers, 1954).

To add further writings would not have added so much quality but quantity - and would have made the production of the volume too expensive. Quotations from the additional material, however, will be used for the following comments.

6.2 Diagnostic Aspects - Psychopathology

The diagnosis "Paranoid Schizophrenia" had already been made by the physicians having treated Mr. T. before he was referred to Ibadan. The symptoms noticed and observations made during his stay at the University College Hospital Ibadan in 1970, at the follow-up visits in 1971 and 1972, and in the letters written by Mr. T. to the author up to the present time, have confirmed the diagnosis.

The fundamental or primary psychopathological signs and symptoms, Bleuler's Four A's (Solomon & Patch, 1969), are present and can be recognized in the writings of Mr. T.

Associative Disturbances are frequent and examples are indicated in the annotations. Condensation of thought, alliteration, repetition and bizarre formulation are exemplified in the modified provervs quoted in his letters:

"Everyone seems to make me a laughing stock or a stepping stone" and: "I will not like my life to be dribbled, even by old associates, as a football, or a ladder and a stepping stone for some others". In some instances it is difficult to decide if an expression like "Touch light" (for torch light) should be interpreted as distortion, neologism, or misspelling. This also applies to the statement: "These peculiar shawdows (sic) or images of objects ...", or: "this move on helpless innoncents (sic)", "I take node (sic) of side effects ...", "... someone ... unirating in a squatting pot or pan", "Earlier when I toned (sic) to Radio Congo ...".- "I urgently need to see you by mid November. Please make this date a date line for me" is a typical example of alliteration. Sometimes Mr. T. is using oldfashioned expressions like "gain said" and "by dint of" for the more common 'deny' and 'by force of'.

Items listed in one of his letters give the impression of loose or automatic associations: "You can imagine such awful objects like excretas, snakes, monkeys, rats, giant rats, female nakedness, skulls, shabby hair, coffins, dishes, soiled males, graves, bones, appearances of the dead, decaying objects, fishes, fowls, pigs, slaughtered meat, huts, buildings in progress, money, cars, lorries, flowers, seas, and figures of people, and the belief by most people that I like particular groups or classes of people". Peculiar formulations are frequent like: "... the ... Government failed ... to explain to me the Ego-function since I am not symbiotically benefitting from the society."

Autism is recognizable in Mr. T.' writings. The contents of the writings are frequently derived from hallucinatory and delusional experiences. In many parts Mr. T.'s thinking is autistic in so far as he has developed a private personal world which he presents in several variations, included in this volume, and in his later letters and scripts of which only few excerpts can be quoted. Mr. T., though, has by no means completely withdrawn into his private, delusional world. He is preoccupied by it, and therefore his communications with the real world might be somewhat disturbed and diminished. But he has still been able to continue with his work and to raise a family. He can also rather easily be distracted from his private world and instigated to collect factual information as e.g. on his MENKA tribe. The modest development of autistic symptons might be characteristic for an African patient.

Affective Incongruity can also be recognized throughout his writings. Frequently Mr. T. reports on terrible and frightening experiences with either a rather flat and blunted affect, or in a humorous or even witty way.

Ambivalence is obvious in the contradictory interpretations of his experiences. On one hand he is absolutely convinced of the reality of his persecutory ideas and other delusions. But on the other hand he always has been and still is "seeking treatment and advice (which) ... a patient needs and which may not be near him where he lives", be it from traditional healers, or from western trained medical doctors. For this purpose he has traveled many thousand miles, wants to come to Germany or Great Britain, and already has spent large amounts of money. "My mind apart from being scorched by psychosis as you term it has been totally demoralised and as such I need to consult you ...". He refers to "... this illness (which) made me to change my natural inclinations and is very dangerous to my health ..." but also writes "It is difficult for a man to stand a vast number of spirits...". He knows "When I tell those things to people... they call me a mad man..." but still continues referring to persecutory ideas: "Even my nearest neighbours are deeply consented to suffering me by this method... (and) I hear people hum and make unusual sounds behind me which only poison me".

He is aware that his "... own way of mannerisms have attracted public attention..." but on the other hand states to see "... now that this is not hallucination as some people may say and that it is not from bodily emotions nor from family background or failures in life but what happens is that some of the friends ... have been and are very avaricious, jealous and full of sexy inclinations...".

Mr. T. is very much preoccupied with his various experiences of hallucinations and delusions, but he still continues his work, raises his growing family and trusts the doctor who has been treating him many years ago: "I will rely on you to advise me on this (voices telling him to go to Great Britain) because God can speak to people in various ways... it is only you who can help me through this fix."

Accessory or secundary symptoms are present in the writings almost everywhere and in great variety.

Auditory hallucinations, generally considered the most common symptoms, are described frequently in Mr. T.'s writings. They occur in divers forms, as noises (akoasms) like grunts, hummings, or sounds, or as voices speaking words, phrases, or sentences, mostly in his own "...dialect i. e. MENKA.." (although) in his vicinity only the patient and his wife are present, or in English. "I heard people speaking to me in the distant, using mixed expressions in my native dialect and English and relate their talking about things concerning me and about people I know; this is so strange to me because my tribesmen are not living in the environment I live."

The noises and voices come from a distance, or are nearby, or originate in his own body: "Distant voices and near ones still commenting on my activities"; "Distinct or clear voices of persons wilfully disturbing me in the office and around the premisses I live, and this brings a sort of psychological warfare in my mind and body"; "The commanding voices came from the roof of my house..."; "I often hear echoes or sounds as of drumming, breaking of wood, etc. in my skull"; "All the scraping dominated by speaking voices within my body...".

Écho de la pensée occurs frequently: "My mind, actions, house have been made like a television where all information is relayed, or cast, by means of dreams, reflection, shadows, shouts, and echoes from people, and other sensational feelings"; "As I write this, every one here knows it, and some echoe back to me what I have written".

Information is withdrawn from his mind and voices are forcing words onto him: "I noted the voices of someone... forcing words out of my heart or throat saying: - vice president"; "Why fetch information from me and add bad thoughts into my mind without my concern?"

Voices comment on or repeat his thoughts, words, and actions. "Whenever I read or say something, some other people around will say 'fraud' or ... will only hum"; "I can not tell why the public should dramatize the Play by action and constant repetition of some words and expressions"; "Kiel is a place and address of my doctor. As often as I write to him using the address people around or even far away start commenting on this name".

What is said by the voices differs widely: "The voices are ... very humiliating and untasteful to a suffering mind..."; "... one of the voices said that I would be taught sex... but I did not experience much about it"; "... those mysterious voices were predicting my flight to Great Britain to do medicine..."; "Many names of places in my own tribe, and also names of persons old and new, or even dead, are constantly repeated to my hearing, and on enquiry, no one can own up. Such (experiences) are not encouraging".

Visual Hallucinations often appear in the form of shadows or images: "There are other forms of shadows of impersonifications usually, during which human figures in the form of shadows are seen, and humming and murmuring voices are... heard in the neighbouring houses or (in the) vicinity"; "Reflection of images of persons and articles some of which I know and others strange in appearance"; the "vision of cars is very common with me since I fell ill"; "I noted a rolling mouvement in my skull and as I looked my eyes were attracted to the floor where I noted a black snake crawling".

Tactile Hallucination frequently are experienced in combination with hallucinations of other sensory modalities: "While resting in bed, I noted someone actually hitting my skull, and the echoe blared through my ears and I recognized a face of a man". Mr. T. reports further: "I usually feel some mouvement in my brain and sometimes ... painful scraping of the inner walls of my chest, something dripping like blood or water down the walls of my chest".

Feelings of bodily change are described repeatedly: "Some (of such groups of beings) cause acute pains or sensations either in the brain, eyes, chest, or belly, and the consequence of this is the harming of the mind and body"; "Around my waist I experience an inflammation of the walls of this region which ... heats my waist ... going through my vertebral column into my brain ... one of the spirits pierced through my body and scraped round my waist causing great pains and introducing itself to be one Dr. Nasah, and said he was operating me and that he had come from America to see me because I was ill".

Olfactory Hallucinations are not mentioned expressively, but frequent references to excreta being put on his head and elsewhere could indicate the experience of hallucinatory bad smells.

No allusions to Gustatory Hallucinations have been found in Mr. T.'s writings.

Paranoid Ideas and Delusions of different types pervade many parts of Mr. T.'s scripts.

Delusions of persecution are prominent: "I am being persecuted by some prominent personalities or groups of people in this country"; "The people who do this have their reasons which I think must be backed by some members of our Government".

He read on "Solomon the Wise... (in) the Plain Truth Magazines about his wisdom during his reigns and how he ended his last days horribly. How this was later translated by the population ... at the time I was afflicted at Kumba on the 20/3/68 at 8 p.m. prompt. The rummours throughout the vicinity that it was because of my READINGS that Solomon Tandeng Muna (see chapter on the MENKA) was nominated Prime Minister of West Cameroon. Hence their beliefs about position and a favouritism on my part".

"Some people who are jealous might have done this to obstruct me from getting what was bright before me"; "Whereever I go agents are behind me"; "The actions of certain people make me believe that some people have been reading my thoughts and actions. This makes me look so suspisiously on some people I know".

Besides being persecuted by people, agents, or politicians, Mr. T.'s delusions include religious ideas and traditional beliefs: "... some aspects of religion are connected with my illness..." and therefore, he wants to be sent "to London to a Catholic psychiatrist after your examination"; "Spirits are wicked beings ... as the Bible describes an incidence of possession of a child by seven bad spirits ... which entered the body of the child, tore his flesh, scraped it, pinned it, and he fell down, cried and rolled himself on the ground and foamed from the mouth until Christ came to his aid".

"I was told by the spirit which said it had command of me for the whole day that I was still a child and my eyes were not yet opened for me to see them who were at the time plentiful"; "... early during this catastrophe in Kumba some of those spirits told me that the snake:

(1) reads information from my books,
(2) can see many, many miles away,
(3) can read one's thoughts.

And ... our local ... society ... want me to sex a woman before this trick/ witchcraft would be given to me".

Quite a number of Mr. T.'s paranoid experiences are concerned with sex, sometimes connected with the feeling of bodily change: "Some cold hands used to touch my private part. Gradually a sort of numbness developed in this part and sensitiveness declined"; "... frequent occurence of nakedness of people both male and female"; "Some especially the sex minded ones, ask me in a hidden manner to have sex with many women"; "I dreamed of having a sex act with a child (N. B. All through this illness, beginning from Kumba ... it had been centred around love and money)"; "I dreamed as I was in a congregation where the priest taught old ladies sex...".

"Just of recent when I lost my mother on the 17. 2. 1979, the gloomy scene on sex occured, and this was carried out by spritual suppression at night. I often saw the nakedness of women and some figures lying by myself or wife or on my bed. You can imagine that this is really Satanic worriness, and it has a tremendous effect on the personality of a person as well as (on) his mind ... There are many women in the neighbourhood who talk very loudly on the situation regarding sex and friends. They often make me to think much about other people and at the same time they assassinate my thoughts and actions".

"Sometime later I heard a lot of slangs ... and it all revealed to me that all was connected to sex".

Other events described by Mr. T. have a more illusionary character as actions of people, or circumstances, perceived in reality are interpreted as having a special meaning: "I have noticed a lot of instances from pedestrians, congregations, people in a market, shops, offices, etc., and their reactions recall their knowledge of the situation i. e. thoughts or actions reading, or what I may term espionage"; "... there is a sort of relay race by any means or form by a set trying to contact some former people I had known"; "... the constant repetition of (the) same symbolic gestures ... ".

"My nearest neighbours ... actually repeat the odd sounds, words, expressions, and names or actions that were performed by spirits before I fell ill ..."; "... most people have unfaithfully claim(ed) to be suffering from this type of illness ... I wonder how they get such information if actually Telepathy was not or is not the Media to link or receive information ... secreteley ... ".

"These people are able to read my thoughts, actions and have the ability to trap (sic - probably word contraction of 'tap' and 'trap') information from my past life, my books, family circle, friends... "; "... feelings and reactions are cast back to you and you recognize them"; "These people often follow me wherever I go ... they follow me by secret means which are above my imagination and I only realise this on my return home during which I hear some voices commenting on the things I did or saw at home"; ; Consequently I deduce that this is a human movement aimed at debarring me from any progress in life ..."; (... these activities) "... are taken by people to suffer my life and debar me from studies and progress, but to use me to educate themselves, get wealthy, or good husbands, and climb up to the tops"; "All these odd and unwanted images sceneries, sharp disturbing impulses and noices (sic) from people which are draining the mind and putting into it unnecessary thoughts and other unbecoming phenomena, worsen conditions of poisoned environment ...".

Sometimes feelings of Depersonalization occur as results of hallucinatory and delusional experiences: "Most people now pretend as though they are suffering from this illness and walk on the same path like me because they can read my thoughts"; or even more direct: "My mind is not mine nor my actions but those of other people".

Grandiose Ideas are the alternative consequence originating from the pathological experiences. Everyone in the country is informed about his life: "The story of my sufferings is known throughout the country"; "The story about my health has spread all over the country and everywhere I go; signs and symptoms of the illness are reflected onto me. The situation is so complicated that more patience from you will discover something new ... in the field of medical science concerning the causes or symptoms of that major mental disease.

You will be doing bad to yourself, my own health and to the world if you fail to hear more information about my health from me".

"The first (report) I had given you has caused a widespread alarm and agitation directed towards me ... by constant repetition everywhere ... because ... copies were given to our regional Broadcasting station ... Some people have read (it) ... or do get it by a supernatural medium and often reflect it back onto a mind that is not yet cured ...".

"All these factors are in connection with environmental and occupational diseases which are man borne diseases as stipulated in U. N. O. Bulletins or World Health Organization's ... There is some sort of social, interstate and intertribal politics interwoven with this issue ..."; " ... any positive or negative reaction accruing from such bad citizens can easily be identified by me"; "Something ... was performed on my head by spirits ... connecting me to many persons by magic threads ... that my pictures would be seen all over the world"; "I do a lot of work, day and night, for so many people. If I read, think, travel, eat, speak, etc. I am doing it for the so many concerned without seeing them for many miles away"; "My name, family and relatives have been projected and we are known everywhere in the country";

"There has been a psychodrama on my part throughout the country. It is still going on now, still, openly by people and by spirits too ... by your own diagnosis 'Psychosis paranoid type'. The condition has developed from one stage to another until the last stage is overdue. Another type of madness has been added to it and that is 'Megalomania' ... it may be another form of development".

6.3 Psychodynamic Aspects

More difficult than a case presentation and a description of psychopathological phenomena, both being attempted in previous sections, would be the psychodynamic interpretation of the dreams, the information available and the observations made.

Not very much is known of Benedict Nta Tanka's childhood and family background. He was born in 1943 as the third of five children to a poor farmer, then about 30 years old, and his senior wife about four years younger than her husband. Living in the traditional way, the family included a junior wife and a third wife, left to the father by a deceased brother. The family belong to a small tribe in the South Western Province of Cameroon, the MENKA.

There was only limited contact to those parts of the country influenced by European colonization and Western ways of life. Mr. T.'s parents tilled the land for subsistence farming earning a little money by palmtree products. Their life was governed by "native laws and customs" examples of which are given in a previous chapter. The parents with their children joined the Catholic faith, possibly when they decided to send their son Benedict to the mission school.

Mr. T. was the first and only of their children to complete elementary school and to study for the higher school examinations which to take he was prevented, according to his own opinion, by his illness. He felt and is still feeling demands made upon him according to both traditional and "modern" ways of life. His development was formed and influenced by traditional and by Western customs.

After leaving school, Mr. T. joined the Government service as a clerk in the Education Office where he is still employed. His intentions to study part-time, besides his work, to advance further in life as many of his friends did were interrupted in 1968 by the onset of his illness. After several periods of sick-leave, the last one in 1974, he has been able, though, to continue with his job but was not able to resume his studies, a severe blow to his self-confidence.

In 1969, at the age of 26, Mr. T. took a 15-year old wife according to native law and custom selected for him by his family. They were married in church two years later and the marriage was recognized by the Government in 1972. Five children were born to his wife and him, the first one in 1970, the last one so far in 1979.

Little is known about Mr. T.'s relationship with his father or his siblings. According to one of his recent letters his mother died in February 1979. In the letter the information on his mother's death was followed by a description of a dream with a "gloomy scene on sex" quoted earlier.

Considering Mr. T.'s reference to sexual activities in his different writings, one is impressed by the predominance of critical or negative attitudes. It is open to conjecture if this is a result of his days in a mission school or a consequence of restrictive rules of his tribe according to his descriptions. There is one positive note on sex, in a letter from 1975, in which he calls it "a wonderful experience" in the beginning, whereas the ending of the paragraph again shows a doubtful attitude: " ... one of the voices said that I would be taught sex in a certain place here in our country but I did not experience much about it. But from September 1974 I noticed a most striking and wonderful experience in which I saw women showing me their nakedness. Some just move naked past me, some open their legs accross my face and I see their sexual organs and ... all sorts of actions of sex were shown to me ... for about two weeks ... You can therefore imagine the thoughts of my mind and the position of my moral character ... Sex is not well taught here as in Europe or other well educated areas. Cameroon is a country that has gone through many colonial masters and the different people have (a) different outlook on sexual affairs... Most Cameroonians have a wrong conception on sex, they misinterprete it and it is highly valued for fortune, education, protection etc... But there are people of certain tribes which have very strict traditions on sex and in olden times and even now cannot have sex until they are married and their purpose for this is not for enjoyment but to raise up a family... Some of us who have been brought up by the traditional and Christian way find it difficult to yield to the needs of the girls or women as society demands... I am suffered in a psychological and supernatural way because of this. The society is trying to influence our traditions especially on sex."

It might be relevant that sexual matters were rarely mentioned in the original writings of Mr. T. written in or before 1970. A distinct inhibition of sexual feelings was assumed, possibly indicating a defence mechanism. In the further writings after 1974 sexual contents became more frequent. However, since he wrote those first reports on his illness, Mr. T. has become a married man and the father of five children. Perhaps the original defence mechanism could be overcome and was given up.

Certainly, cultural conflicts must have been influential in the personality development of Benedict Tanka. This is illustrated by his dreams and psychotic experiences in which traditional spirits as well as modern technology play their parts.

Simenauer (1961) in his article on the Oedipus conflict in Bantu patients from East Africa emphasizes the strong influence of tribal customs and pressures which are acting also on urbanized patients often causing "severe conflict situations and psychopathological signs as they are typical for the 'man of two worlds' ". The African ways of rearing children, at least in some tribes, might not only contribute to an easy solution of the Oedipal conflict but might also help to prevent severe regression and "falling into pieces of the ego" in schizophrenic patients.

Fortes (1959) emphasizes the importance of the concept of "fate" and "destination" in Westafrican religion explaining it by the very close child-parent relationship. The experience of "destination" permeates Mr. T.'s writings. The rarity of reference to his relationship with his parents may be of importance.

Psychoanalytical studies in different Westafrica tribes (Parin et al. 1963; 1971) illustrate remarkable differences of e.g. child rearing practices, consequent personality formation and neurotic defence mechanisms, warning against applying research results of one ethnical group to other groups. Staewen and Schoenberg (1970) also warn against "superficial, unwise and often prejudicial generalizations" of psychodynamic observations. Thus, one has to be very careful when considering observations from other tribes. However, in trying to understand Mr. T.'s experiences, the concept of a "normal paranoid" (Parin et al. 1971) seems helpful. In the authors opinion, "normal" paranoid feelings are both more prominent and better integrated in Africans than in Europeans. The "paranoid" of Mr. T. certainly has overgrown the "normal" level; nevertheless, he is able to live with it. Descriptions of the authors seem to apply well to Mr. T.:

"Aggressive tendencies are easily shifted, have no tendency to centre upon one object and an accumulation of aggressive tendencies only happens incompletely ... the tendency is modest to fight the cruel object in the real world" (Parin et al. 1971).

A few notions may conclude this section:

- It is remarkable how dream contents and psychotic experiences are overlapping.
- In both dreams and psychotic occurances many people already dead figure prominently.
- Members of Mr. T.'s parental as well as of his own family do not appear often in the dreams and in the psychotic events.
- Some meanings of both dreams and psychotic experiences are difficult for a foreigner to comprehend. Intensive studies and additional

informations obtained recently from Mr. T. have helped to understand his writings better.

To study psychodynamic aspects in Mr. T.'s writings in greater depth would require not only more and more specific information on his background, but also an psychoanalyst with expert experience in cultural anthropology. Perhaps, this volume can serve as research material. One purpose of the publication would be achieved when it could stimulate further studies in this and other fields.

6.4 Follow-up and Therapeutic Aspects 1974 to 1979

The history of Mr. T.'s disease can be divided into two periods. The first period begins with the onset of the psychosis in March 1968 and ends with a letter written by Mr. T. early in 1973 to the editor then still being in Ibadan. This period is covered in the case notes in a previous section. The three reports by Mr. T. published fully belong to this period. After Mr. T. did not keep an appointment in Ibadan for 1973, the possibility of further contact with him was not anticipated, and the original manuscript was completed in the early months of this year before the editor left Ibadan, and publication was intended.

However, when the editor visited Ibadan in 1974 a letter of Mr. T. was waiting for him. Another letter was forwarded to his home address. Both letters were asking for help and urgently requesting attention. An intensive correspondence developed, comprising 43 letters of more than 140 pages, written in irregular intervals, at some times with increasing frequency not related to the infrequent replies of the editor. Mr. T. wrote 6 letters in 1974, 8 in 1975, 14 in 1976, 3 in 1977, none between 20 September 1977 and 12 April 1979, date of the first letter of a new series of 12 in 1979.

These 43 communications, including further lengthy descriptions of his old and new experiences, and replies to three questionnaires of the editor, are the source for the second period, the follow-up from early 1974 until the end of 1979.

Each time the letters became more frequent in 1974, in 1976 and in 1979, form and content of the letters indicated an exacerbation of the psychosis. The prescription of appropriate neuroleptic medication on two occasions was followed by an improvement of the condition recognizable in the letters, and acknowledged by Mr. T.

Despite temporary detoriations of his health, Mr. T. was able, except for a short sick-leave in late 1974, to continue with his work regularly, whilst he was given light duties and was relieved from typing. To his chagrin he was not promoted during the 12 years since the illness had started.

Pharmacotherapy, reported in the case history, was the main line of treatment during the in-patient care at Ibadan in 1970. Chlorpromazine alone was not effective but under Trifluperazine all psychotic symptoms disappeared: "... speaking voices within my body lasted for three months and began to die down after I had treatment at the Hospital."; "... there was some sort of break from this unusual illness after my treatment in Ibadan in 1970 and the subsequent consultations and treatment in 1971 and 1972".

After discharge a relapse occured when the drug was not available. It subsided after Triperidol was prescribed at the follow-up visit in 1971. At his last visit to Ibadan in 1972 he was well. Pimozid was prescribed and a supply was given to last until his next visit scheduled for June 1973 which Mr. T. was not able to keep. Apparently a further relapse occured after the drug was finished: "These objects . . . were not frequent until early September 1973 when this symptom reappeared again until the present moment of my writing these notes" on 9 July 1974, "... I have been buying the drugs prescribed by you ... with the exception of Orap forte which is not found in Cameroon...".

In reply to many letters requesting help Mr. T. at first was advised to seek psychiatric treatment in his country. He experienced these attempts as not very successful: "I have some argumentatative tendency towards the new psychiatrist because he has not studied the case very closely as you did. He asks no questions to me"; "I have moved to almost every town in this country seeking treatment" (1974); "I refuse to be hospitalized in Yaounde because I have noticed that the more I am there, the more I will get miserable" (1975); "The local doctors have failed to tell me what is wrong" (1975); "I have gone around the entire country seeking treatment with Native Doctors, medical Doctors, both private and Government but have not seen no better for these nine years. I have spent over 2 million (C. F. A.) francs" (approximately $ 12.000) (1975); "I have been to Yaounde for about twelve times since September 1973 up til now spending over £ 200 all on tablets and transport" (1976).

Also his Head of Department and his doctor wrote to request help from the editor, because "Mr. Tanka has much faith on your treatment since he responded so much to it" and "Since he lost touch of you, he has had severe attacks that none of the Doctors here has been able to remedy". Complying with the repeated requests, after correspondence with his doctor in Cameroon, a supply of Pimozid (Orap Janssen) was sent to Buea provided by the manufacturers.

After starting to take the drug again, Mr. T.'s condition improved once more: "I am writing to thank you for the recent batch of medicines you sent to me through Dr. B. .. There is nothing doubting that you are my good Samaritan as far as my health is concerned" (Dec. 1976). The three letters sent in 1977 did not show any pathological signs. There were no letters in 1978.

In his next letter of 12 April 1979, written 19 months after the last one and about nine months after the supply of drugs should have been exhausted, Mr. T. again asks for medical help. The subsequent letters clearly indicate a gradual detoriation of his health and a reappearance of the former symptoms. After some correspondence in which the possibilities of a journey of Mr. T. to Germany for personal consultation were discussed, it was decided this time to prescribe Penfluridal (Semap Janssen) and a supply was sent to Mr. T. provided again by the manufacturers. In the following letter, written after having taken three tablets of 20 mg each in weekly intervals, improvement was recognizable. This impression increased in the five letters written until Dec. 1979.

Treatment from a distance is considered of doubtful effectiveness and problematic in regard of professional standards. Nevertheless, the very special circumstances, the repeated favourable results and the profound knowledge of the patient's illness and reactions could, as a rare exception, justify the procedure. Mr. T. writes: "Your services both old and new are still very helpful to me now especially that you have to put me on medication from your end".

Psychotherapy accompanied the basic pharmacotherapy throughout. The base of the supportive, councilling, explanatory, advisory and reassuring psychotherapy was the strong therapeutic relationship which developed between Mr. T. and the writer during many intensive interviews at Ibadan and was reinforced by the correspondence lasting more than five years.

The importance of the written communication with the therapist is frequently mentioned by Mr. T.: "It gives me much pleasure to write to you as often as possible"; "I am glad to take another turn to write to you about my problem"; "I feel to write to you often (because) I believe that you stand in a better position to listen to my problem"; "I have revealed my mind to you through conversation with you and through writings especially that story of my illness".

The intensive feelings of Mr. T. for his therapist appear repeatedly in his writings, the therapist sometimes being included in delusional experiences: "Most say your report about me was false or that I bribed you"; "Girls have grouped themselves in gangs, one says I am Dr. Boroffka, the others say I am that etc."; "How I wish that you are sent to Cameroon"; "If your Government does not approve that I see my loving Dr. B. this will have an adverse effect on my mind"; "I am very glad and thankful to My God to see you have such a keen interest in me"; "... you are the only person to get me out of the burning bush ...".

The scientific interest of the therapist certainly has contributed to his willingness to spend time and effort on the patient; but it also might have increased the therapeutic efficacy, and has reinforced the therapist's rôle as "participant observer" (Sullivan, 1953). The therapist's letters written between 1974 and 1979, show a basic attitude: The therapist in his replies took absolutely serious everything the patient had written.

It would be unrealistic to assume the few letters sent by the therapist over the years could have had a major psychotherapeutic effect. But they have kept Mr. T. on the one thing which has helped him besides the drugs: To write about his experiences to somebody of whose attention he felt certain. This activity, a form of self-therapy, might have contributed to the favourable course of his illness (Wing, 1977).

Frequently the author has found it helpful to request from suitable patients to write autobiographies. This proved advantagious in two ways. In a busy clinic in Africa with a scarcity of psychiatric services it is helpful to have part of the history written down by the patient himself. Originally, this had been the author's main objective. But later he found that the patients' writing down their life histories seems to have a therapeutic function which could be explained that it serves as a cathartic outlet. By writing down his problems a patient already makes an effort to overcome them and to gain distance towards them.

Still, psychotherapy by correspondence is at most the second best way; therefore it is understandable that Mr. T. wants to visit the therapist and consult him personally again. He has expressed this wish in many letters since 1976: "... the urgent desire to see you personally..."; "I wish ... there should be no hesitation in letting me come over there..."; "I am now totally weak and stupid and no great man or other authority can view this urgent to send me to you as soon as possible or else I would have been there ever since"; "If only you can strike at the point at once for me to come ..." (1976); "...I wish to ask you to tell me as soon as possible by the next mail the exact time and date I will be in Germany for my treatment"; "I was delighted with the packet of medicine you enclosed and I hope this will help me before I meet you. . ."(1979). Specific travel arrangements are requested and proposals made in the subsequent letters. Nobody has been found to pay the cost of the journey what had to be explained to the patient once and again.

Preparations for the Publication of his edited and annotated writings have been followed by Mr. T. with keen interest. Since 1970 he has favoured the publishing of his reports. In his letters he frequently enquires about the book: "... the book you said you will make on me from the material you got from me... how far have ... (the assessors) gone with this work?"; "I am also glad to learn that you are up and doing about the printing of the story"; "What about that our book? I am still writing more about my illness"; "I hope progress is on that book..."; "You will get more from me to build up that book"; "... the most interesting part of the story is the play which I thought would form a second part of the first one with you. But I will not be able to do it as you have asked me to stop it"; "I am sorry about your inability to have those notes or stories on myself publicated. However, I know I brought them to you to help you understand the background of my problem of health. An advice from one Reverend Father ... was that I should preserve it for the future... So I believe since the issues presented are very thrilling and teaching to the medically inclined people or even people with different inclinations to life, we are going to be successful in printing a large book from the issues... I think all my own correspondences to you and even yours to me ... will form material for more chapters or scenes"; "Please, sir, forget about the recent questionnaire ... and build your facts right from the time I consulted you in Ibadan on Friday 25th September 1970. According to your diagnosis, this type of illness 'Psychosis paranoid type' has different stages and now the last of the stages is overdue. Accordingly from my mouvements and long experience for over twelve years on this illness it is concluded that it has social and political effects and another characteristic has been added to it by the populations of this Nation. This state is known as 'Megalomania' which is a form of madness that gives a person the idea that he is important and very great which only buoys (instead of 'boils' - neologism) down to headiness and stubbornness"; "I hope you should not hurry over the question of publishing the book about me because more information will be given to you before publication". It seems material for a second volume may soon be at hand...

Traditional Healers were consulted frequently by Mr. T. The word for them in the MENKA language is Verikanbeong. Since 1972 he has consulted

Mr. Joseph Empah, a MENKA, "very famous but unlizensed"; Mr. Lucas Mokam, belonging to the METTA tribe (as the former Prime Minister of West Cameroon), Mr. Raymond Tantang, a BAMUMBU, and Mr. Fokam.

On previous experiences with traditional healers Mr. T. wrote in 1976: "Before meeting you in Ibadan, ... I had already consulted some three native herbalists here and on my return I also met other three. Each one of them gave his views which I must tell you on arrival but the impetus put forth by the general public has food for thought as to the face that my mouvements were/are being watched, and perhaps such native doctors might have been approached somehow by such 'guides' either not used for an act useful to the public... at the expense of my health which they themselves pretend to believe that my own feelings and complaints on my nerves were false".

The descriptions of the activities of traditional healers in his reports are worthwhile to be studied. Their methods might be effective in conditions in which the knowledge of social and psychological factors of the patient and his environment are crucial but may accomplish less in cases like that of Mr. T. when a major psychosis is present. Mr. T.'s long journeys to different traditional healers at different places located far apart and not belonging to his own or a related tribe, typical for to-days situation of mobility in Westafrica, makes it doubtful if the traditional healers consulted were familiar with the life circumstances of our patient originating from a small tribe living off the main roads.

Sometimes Mr. T.'s narrative indicates that the traditional healers encourage paranoid projections by accusing spirits or 'witches' of causing illness and especially mental illness (Asuni, 1968). According to the author's observations (Boroffka, 1973a) traditional healers rarely enquire about the patient's background or family even of clients who have come from far away.

Remarkable in all references to treatment is the similarity of the patient's emotional attitude towards consultations of traditional healers and of western trained physicians; there is no guarantee for help from either one. Mr. T.'s experiences with traditional healers should make one cautious of the view, being fashionale nowadays (Singer, 1977), that therapy provided by traditional healers is always superior to western medicine in Africans suffering from mental disorders.

6.5 Transcultural Aspects

Transcultural psychiatry, started in times past by Kraepelin (1904) and continued by many scholars since (Wittkower et al. 1956 - 1979; Pfeiffer, 1971; Kiev, 1972), has been especially interested in the comparison of mental disorders in relationship to cultural differences. Cooperation of psychiatry with other scientific fields stimulated research. Close collaboration with anthropology has been most successful (Wittkower & Dubreuil, 1971). The aim of comparative as part of transcultural psychiatry has been a better understanding of the aetiology of mental disorders and of "mental patients ... regardless of the culture in which they live" (Sartorius, 1979).

Epidemiological studies on representative numbers of patients or populations can provide percentile figures as answers to questions of occurance, frequency, symptomatology, or typical course and outcome of special disorders, like paranoid schizophrenia, in relation to certain cultures.

The study of many patients (e.g. Boroffka, 1973b), necessarily superficial in regard of the single case, can be supplemented by case studies, having gone somewhat out of fashion, like this one devoted to a single patient and his background. In so far the publication of Mr. T.'s writings together with editorial comments and supplements is intended as a contribution to transcultural psychiatry, besides offering to the interested reader a unique opportunity to observe at first hand the working of an "African mind in health and disease" (Carothers, 1954).

Some authors (Carothers, 1954), quoting earlier studies on African patients, held the opinion that paranoid schizophrenia and especially pronounced, systematized delusions are rare or absent in illiterate societies. Pfeiffer (1971) reviewed the more recent literature and found structured delusions less frequent in the lower social strata, mostly illiterate, of many traditional societies. Lambo (1953; 1954), though, found paranoid psychoses as frequent in Africans, unrelated to the grade of western education, than elsewhere. In 1.490 admissions in Lagos/Nigeria (Boroffka, 1973b) almost 30% of the schizophrenic patients belonged to the paranoid type; about one half of all the patients admitted were illiterate; the distribution of diagnoses was not related to literacy.

Mr. T.'s writings show a fully developed, systematized, fairly well structured paranoid or delusional system in a patient originating from an illiterate peasant family, which lived far away from urbanized and westernized areas, and had become Christian only when the patient was to join a mission school. Mr. T. was the very first, and for a long time the only one, in his family who had the opportunity to go to school: "... being the only child who can read and write in my own family, and again (in) my own tribe since colonial days of the German people and even later by the English people... there was no educated people here; (the tribe) is not represented in both, civil service and private sectors of the country's administration and other commercial services, nor has it ever had any representation in the Regional ... or Federal Government ... the MENKA people speak MENKA which has not yet been written down in books...".

The writings of the first literate member of an illiterate society, of which he gives a vivid description, might help the reader to form his own answer to the question if there are more similarities or dissimilarities in the symptomatology of paranoid schizophrenia between this case and cases from western culture. Many classical symptoms of the condition are recognizable in Mr. T.'s writings. Annotations referring to them had to be restricted in order not to become too cumbersome. There is hardly a paragraph without the indication of a schizophrenic symptom.

Many authors, recently reviewed by Corin & Murphy (1979), have related the frequency of mental disorders including schizophrenia to an increasing degree of westernization. Fascinating observations in this respect have been made by Fortes & Mayer (1969) who had the unique opportunity to live with a small tribe in rural Ghana twice, the two periods of study divided by thirty years. At their second stay the authors found a distinct increase of the number of mental patients in the population compared with the first stay, which observation they related hypothetically to the increase of westernization during this time.

Little can be contributed to the question of a possible increase of mental disorders by the study of a single case. However, considering factors possibly influencing Mr. T.'s psychosis, cultural change, the clash of two cultures with differing value systems (Staewen & Schoenberg, 1970), rather than the increasing westernization itself might have played a part in it.

Mr. T.'s report of a dream in which he is pursued by "... foes speaking METTA/MOGHAMO..." (META a language group north-north-west of Bali, the MOGHAMO living at Bafawchu in the NGEMBA tribal area; both belong to the WIDEKUM group and are close neighbours of the MENKA. - Westermann & Bryan, 1952) and the fact that a politician, Solomon Tandeng Muma, figuring prominently in Mr. T.'s writings, belong to the same tribe, could suggest an interrelation of tribal rivalry and antagonism on the political level.

Fortes & Mayer (1969) and many other authors have observed that schizophrenia can easily be diagnosed by western standards, but very often takes a much more benign course.

The course of Mr. T.'s disease has so far also been rather favourable and has differed from the course this illness usually takes in patients from industrialized countries. Mayer-Gross (1969) writes "in the majority of cases, acute paranoid psychoses are the beginning of a chronic illness... Remissions after a longer paranoid psychosis are usually approximations to a social adjustment". The first part of the statement applies to Mr. T.'s case: his illness started as an acute paranoid psychosis which was the beginning of a chronic illness. However, the clinical notes on the two follow-up periods show that his condition has improved remarkably. Mr. T. has been working regularly since his discharge from hospital in 1970, now for more than nine years, and has readjusted himself to social life. This is more than an "approximation to a social adjustment". Few signs of the illness were left at his visit in 1972. Judging from a letter his condition was even more favourable in 1973.

Regular contacts with Mr. T. were maintained by correspondence until the present time (1979). His condition has varied considerably throughout the years, apparently connected with the availability of effective drug maintenance therapy. At four occasions (1971, 1974, 1976, 1979) acute exacerbations of his psychosis have occured and subsided rather immediately after neuroloptic drugs of the Butyrophenone type became again available. Even those episodes have not prevented him from continuing his work, have not required hospitalization, and have not removed him from his social environment.

Of course, this course of the illness could be one of the rare exceptions for which Mayer-Gross (1969) makes an allowance although it would be an extremely rare exception in European or American patients. However, when this course is compared with similar conditions, encountered in African and patients from other developing countries, it is not unusual.

In this context the International Pilot Study on Schizophrenia (WHO, 1973; 1979) must be mentioned. Its main conclusions apply also to a single case as presented here:

- A therapeutic relationship can be formed and maintained for a long period of time between a psychiatrist from Europe and a patient from a country with different cultural and socioeconomic conditions. This makes possible a scientific evaluation and presentation compairable to studies from other countries.
- The diagnostic and psychopathological classification of schizophrenia does not differ from those in countries of other cultures.
- The follow-up of Mr. T.'s illness over almost twelve years agrees with the result of the IPSS (WHO, 1979) that social outcome in patients suffering from schizophrenia very often is more favourable in those from developing countries than in patients from industrialized countries.

6.6. Literary Aspects

There exists a large number of publications on the relationship between art and mental illness. A survey has been published recently (Bader & Navratil, 1979). A certain preference for pictorial or graphic arts can be observed. However, psychiatrists for a long time have been fascinated by either literary quality of the writings of schizophrenic patients, or by psychiatric characteristics in works of literature and/or in the personalities of writers. The latter has produced a wide field of pathographies exemplified in the famous volume by Lange-Eichbaum (1932).

In more recent times also men of letters have been fascinated by writings of schizophrenics with regard to contents and aesthetic qualities. A recent anthology (Kudszus, 1977) brings together articles by psychiatrists and literati.

Autobiographies of schizophrenic patients are at first of clinical interest, as documents of the patient's thinking and feeling, helping the psychiatrist to diagnose a patient, understand his problems better, and thereby finding an effective therapeutic approach more easily.

Autobiographical and other writings of patients were well known to psychiatrists of former times when many schizophrenic patients stayed in hospital for long periods of time. Being so common, there was little interest in publishing those writings, except occasional excerpts in psychiatric textbooks or articles. As a curiosity some autobiographies were published in full by patients on their own expenses. Some such publications of olden times have been reprinted in recent years when general interest in such works increased. An example is the "Cry for Help of a Magnetically Poisened Patient" (Krauss, 1967).

More famous have become Schreber's "Memoirs of my Nervous Illness", a unique volume, which has been reprinted many times (1972; 1973) and has been translated into English (Macalpine & Hunter, 1955). It became well known already soon after it was published over 75 years ago (Schreber, 1903) and has been quoted subsequently in many psychiatric textbooks (Bleuler, Kraepelin, Adolf Meyer, Mayer-Gross et al.) as a history of a paranoid schizophrenia seen from the inside, providing at the same time examples of schizophrenic symptoms of various categories. Schreber's volume became more widely known when Freud (1911) based on it his paper on the origins of paranoia.

Mr. T.'s writings are the first autobiography of an African schizophrenic, or of any patient from outside the western world, to be published. Therefore it seemed adequate to refer to the Schreber case in the subtitle of this book. Mr. T.'s opus has qualities comparable to the "Memoirs..."; it gives the history of a paranoid psychosis from the inside, narrating it in three differend variations, and elaborating on it in the subsequent correspondence. The writings contain many examples of primary and secondary symptoms of schizophrenia. Furthermore, the overlapping and integrating of traditional and western cultural elements are recognizable throughout the volume. Along with Schreber's "Memoirs..." it can serve to compare the course of paranoid schizophrenia without and under the influence of neuroleptic medication.

Mr. T. writes on the Schreber "Memoirs...": "At Ibadan, you showed me a book written by Schreber from your library and the contents were on his health i. e. (a) written account of himself after an illness. I believe you have enough material now and later on will revise it before ... you embark on making a full publication ...".

Besides being a clinical document presenting remarkable features, Mr. T.'s writings exert a strong fascination by its literary characteristics. The unmistakable Westafrican flavour is formed by various influences which include the English Bible and classical literature, contributed by the mission school, the local literature as exemplified by the Onitsha market publications (Beier, 1964, Obiechina, 1971; 1972), and finally characteristics of the writer's own vernacular. Of further significance is the contribution of pidgin English, the essential lingua franca of countries in which scores of different languages and dialects, mutually incomprehensible, are spoken within small territories, as it is the case in Cameroon.

Attention should also be called to a certain poetic quality of Mr. T.'s writings by quoting a few examples. The engaged reader will easily find many more: "For twelve good years of personal efforts you have in vain failed to uncover the secret of my mind"; - "For my own little knowledge, I believe the mind can only be broadened by doing sensible things as laid down by generations gone by"; - "The training, spiritual, intellectual, and physical - that young people receive in the home determines in no small way their destiny for the time and eternity"; - "Well, if I knew all the secrets of the world and the wishes of the people on me ... then I should not be worried"; - "Real distant voices are not only displeasing but a big handicap to my ever green ill-health"; - "This is a melancholy age in Cameroon whereby all things go round on me and I know not why".

6.7 Closing Remarks

After clinical and literary aspects have been dealt with in previous sections, the volume prepared by a physician ought to end by emphasizing that the principal writer, Benedict Nta Tanka, is a patient suffering from experiences, which might be fascinating to the observer but are awful and frightening to him, requiring help and support: "The type of language used is now very common among the people ... their expressions are mostly in my own dialect and very humiliating and untasteful to a suffering mind"; - "You know that this type of illness brings misery when often I am forced into thoughts by voices of people who cannot come out plainly and speak to me ..."; - "... imagine the strains and stresses on my mind and body caused by this for this very long period. Haunting at night is so rampant, even during the day, and such uncouthed people cannot express themselves ... You can understand the aweful situation a weak mind like this will encounter throughout a very long period with sleepless and thoughtful nights"; - "... from the above date, all my friends escaped and were perhaps indoctrinated by a national fraud... I ought to have educated myself fully if I were not interrupted by this wicked act... What are they doing with me now that I roamed to all parts of this country under pains and pressures but no one seems to stop the nonsense..."; - "... they have thrust my family people into smoke, and even friends I had won ... by dint of hard labour... you see that the less favoured people are often tossed up and down in this way"; - "Since this ... was portrayed to me through evil spirits causing dangers to my life, ... this has left the mind always in bewilderment and pains... and the more one stays in the agony for such a long time without a clue, it is not far from one becoming a Lunatic person"; - "... the sufferer feels much pain (more) than the actor who laughs all the time and may not believe the patient"; - "I have tried to resist the impact for eight years but all my efforts have proved a failure (as) my useful time and youth ... has been spoiled ... I find no place in Black Africa to rest and (to) forget my troubles"; - "The last stage of 'psychosis' or this illness has passed over since, and the more the people dramatize it the more miserable I become".

Notwithstanding all his sufferings, Mr. T. continuously is trying to overcome his predicament by, among other activities, his writings: "It gives me such pleasure to write to you as often as possible...". He tries to find explanations for his illness: "... some now realize that my problem was or is true and must have a political motivation... You will now agree with me that this sort of illness is motivated by people through a media in which the spirits actually play the part in order that I who belong not to this group, should not know those burning fires on my head, or it may be I am understudied in an unknown way as psychoanalysis or spiritual ..."; - "... this type of miraculous mouvement ... was caused by our own society and population. So unless (they) ... decide to stop their ungodly mouvement I will never be well no matter how much money I spend because of this ill-health"; - "Our society is still backward and full of envy from emerging youngsters, adults, and tribes and man's life can be tortured or ill-treated in a diversity of ways"; - "The population are looking at myself as a playboy and an insane man for all time"; - "From the onset everything was miraculously performed by spirits, yet in the course of time the menacing actions of spirits died down gradually and gave way to voices of real people which now repeat the actions of the invisible... spirits"; - "Socialism and public interest has a great part to play in addition to the present politics of our society, and love have contributed to this sort of illness although many people will associate it to hereditary and childhood problems"; - "... even now I am only learning to return to normality ..."; - " ... my views ... on the situation ... are a result of careful observations, hard sufferings, and much expenditure"; - "If it is imagination, then it comes contrary to the will and uncalled for. Therefore there must be a source or a lack of a certain hormone in the body"; - "I hope you must take note of the theory of Psychoanalysis and something about thought reading. These are very touching to the mind and have the effect of Psychological Warfare especially when your feelings and actions are cast back to you and you recognize them"; - "I am gaining good grounds about the causes of the illness and those who are likely involved in it"; - "It may be I was the only one hearing these voices because I was possessed or haunted by spirits...".

Through the interest taken by the editor in the reports, Mr. T. develops the conviction that "more patience ... will discover something new ... in the field of medical sciences concerning the causes or symptoms of that major mental disease. You will be doing bad to yourself, my own health, and to the world if you fail to hear more information about my health from me".

Contact with Mr. T. will be kept. "Treatment by correspondence" and by drugs will be continued. A reunion of the patient with the therapist might be possible in the future. But, perhaps, the most decisive part in the course of the events, described in this book, is played by Mr. T.'s writings, turning his life, as it happens in the play, "from a tragedy into the happy ending of a comedy - a triumph of health over disease".

7. REFERENCES

Anderson, E. W.; Trethowan, W. H. (1967): Psychiatry. Second Edition. London: Baillière, Tindall & Cassell.

Asuni, T. (1969): Methods of delivering mental health care. Paper read at a workshop on: The Delivery of Mental Health Care. Kampala: cyclostyled script.

Bader, A.; Navratil, L. (1979): Psychiatrie und Kunst. In: Kisker, K. P. et al. (Eds.): Psychiatrie der Gegenwart Band I, Teil 1; Second Edition. Berlin: Springer-Verlag.

Beier, U. (1964): Public opinion on lovers. Popular Nigerian literature sold in Onitsha market. Black Orpheus No 14. Ibadan: Mbari.

Boroffka, A. (1973a): Management of Madness; Past and Present. Film in colour and with sound. Sandoz (Nigeria) Ltd.

Boroffka, A. (1973b): Mental illness in Lagos: History and admission statistics of the Yaba Mental Hospital from 1907 to 1966. Psychopathologie africaine 9, 405-417.

Carothers, J. C. (1954): The African Mind in Health and Disease. Wld Hlth Org. Monograph. No. 17. Geneva.

Corin, E.; Murphy, H. B. M. (1979): Psychiatric perspectives in Africa. Part I: the Western viewpoint. Transcultural Psychiatric Research Review 16, 147-178

Encyclopaedia Britannica (1973): Articles on:

African Languages	Vol.	1, pp.	312 ff.
Bamileke	"	3, p.	71
Bamum	"	3, p.	72
Bantu Languages	"	3, pp.	135 ff.
Cameroon	"	4, pp.	702 ff.
Tikar	"	21, p.	1146

Fortes, M. (1959): Oedipus and Job in West African Religions. Cambridge: Cambridge University Press.

Fortes, M.; Mayer, D. Y. (1969): Psychosis and Social Change among the Tallensi of Northern Ghana. In: S. H. Foulkes; G. S. Prince (Eds.): Psychiatry in a Changing Society. London: Tavistock Publications.

Freud, S. (1911): Psycho-analytic notes upon an autobiographical account of a case of paranoia (dementia paranoides). In: Collected Papers, 3, 390-467.

Greenberg, J.H. (1955): Studies in African Linguistic Classification. Branford, Conn.: Compass, Box 321.

Kiev, A. (1972): Transcultural Psychiatry. New York: The Free Press.

Kraepelin, E. (1904): Vergleichende Psychiatrie. Zentralblatt fuer Nervenheilkunde und Psychiatrie 27, 433-437.

Krauss, F. (1967): Nothschrei eines Magnetisch-Vergifteten (1852) und Nothgedrungene Fortsetzung meines Nothschrei (1867). Ausgewählt und kommentiert von H. Ahlenstiel; J. E. Meyer (Eds.): Selbstschilderungen eines Geisteskranken. Leverkusen: Bayer.

Kudszus, W. (Ed.) (1977): Literatur und Schizophrenie. Theorie und Interpretation eines Grenzgebietes. Tübingen: Niemeyer und dtv.

Lambo, T. A. (1954): Observations on the Role of Cultural Factors in Paranoid Psychosis among the Yoruba Tribe: a Study in Comparative Psychiatry. M.D. Thesis. Birmingham.

Lambo, T. A. (1955): The role of cultural factors in paranoid psychoses among the Yoruba tribe. J. Ment. Sci. 101, 239-266.

Lange-Eichbaum, W. (1932): The Problems of Genius. New York: Macmillan. Translation of: Genie, Irrsinn und Ruhm; München: Reinhardt 1928.

Macalpine, I.; Hunter, R. A. (1955): Daniel Paul Schreber Memoirs of my Nervous Illness. Translated, Edited, with Introduction, Notes and Discussion. London: WM, Dawson & Sons Ltd.

Marum, E. (1975): A Discussion of some Cultural Issues Relevant to the Case of Benedict Tanka. Manuskript, 5 pages (Personal Communication).

Mayer-Gross, W.; Slater, E.; Roth, M. (1969): Clinical Psychiatry. 3rd Edition. London: Baillière, Tindall & Cassell.

Obiechina, E. (1971): Literature for the Masses. Enugu: Nwankwo-Ifejika & Co. Publishers.

Obiechina, E.N. (1972): Onitsha Market Literature. London, Ibadan, Nairobi: Heinemann.

Parin, P.; Morgenthaler, F.; Parin-Matthèy, G. (1963): Die Weißen denken zu viel. Psychoanalytische Untersuchungen bei den Dogon in Westafrika Zürich: Atlantis.

Parin, P.; Morgenthaler, F.; Parin-Matthèy, G. (1971): Fürchte deinen Nächsten wie dich selbst. Psychoanalyse und Gesellschaft am Modell der Agni in Westafrika. Frankfurt/M.: Suhrkamp.

Pfeiffer, W.M. (1971): Transkulturelle Psychiatrie. Stuttgart: Thieme.

Prince, R. (1960): The use of Rauwolfia for the treatment of psychoses by Nigerian native doctors. Am. J. Psychiat. 117, 147.

Prince, R.; Speed, F. (1963): Were ni - He is a mad man. Film in colour and sound.

Sartorius, N. (1979): Crosscultural Psychiatry. In: Kisker, K.P. et al. (Eds.): Psychiatrie der Gegenwart Band I, Teil 1; Second Edition. Berlin: Springer-Verlag.

Schreber, D.P. (1903): Denkwürdigkeiten eines Nervenkranken. Leipzig: Oswald Mutze.

Schreber, D.P. (1972): Denkwürdigkeiten eines Nervenkranken (1903). Reprint in: Bürgerliche Wahnwelt um Neunzehnhundert. Hrsg. P. Heiligenthal; R. Volk. Wiesbaden: Focus Verlag; reprinted 1973. Mit Aufsätzen von Franz Baumayer.

Schreber, D.P. (1973): Denkwürdigkeiten eines Nervenkranken. Herausgegeben und eingeleitet von S.M. Weber. Frankfurt/M.: Verlag Ullstein GmbH.

Segal, R. (1961): Political Africa. A Who's Who of Personalities and Parties. London: Stevens & Sons, Ltd.

Seligman, C.G. (1961): Races of Africa. 3rd Ed. London: Oxford University Press.

Simenauer, E. (1961): Ödipuskonflikt und Neurosebedingungen bei den Bantu Ostafrikas. Jahrbuch der Psychoanalyse. Band II, 41-62.

Singer, P. (1977): Traditional Healing: New Science or New Colonialism? Essays in Critique of Medical Anthropology. Owerri, New York, London: Conch Magazine Lts. (Publ.)

Solomon, Ph.; Patch, V.D. (Eds.) (1969):
Handbook of Psychiatry. Lange Medical Publications, USA.

Spiess, C.H. (1966): Biographien der Wahnsinnigen. Berlin: Luchterhand.

Staewen, C.; Schoenberg, F. (1970):
Kulturwandel und Angstentwicklung bei den Yoruba Westafrikas. München: Weltforum-Verlag.

Sullivan, H.S. (1953): The Interpersonal Theory of Psychiatry. New York: W. W. Norton & Co. Inc.

Talbot, P.A.; Mulhall, H. (1962):
The Physical Anthropology of Southern Nigeria. A Biometric Study in Statistical Method. Cambridge: University Press.

Vyncke, J. (1957): L'Assistance psychiatrique en Ruanda-Urundi; In: Mental Disorders and Mental Health in Africa South of the Sahara. CCTA Publication No. 35.

Westermann, D.; Bryan, M.A. (1952):
Languages of West Africa; Handbook of African Languages, Part II. London: Oxford University Press for the International African Institute.

Wing, J.K. (1977): Schizophrenie in Selbstzeugnissen; deutsche Übersetzung von "Schizophrenia from Within" (National Schizophrenia Fellowship). In: H. Katschnig (Ed.): Die andere Seite der Schizophrenie: Patienten zu Hause. Fortschritte der Sozialpsychiatrie 2. München: Urban & Schwarzenberg.

Wittkower, E.D. (1969): Perspectives of transcultural psychiatry. Internation J. Psychiat. 8, 811-824.

Wittkower, E.D.; Fried, J. et al. (Eds.) (1956-1979):
Transcultural Psychiatric Research Review. Montréal: McGill-Queen's University Press.

Wittkower, E.D.; Dubreuil, G. (1971):
Reflections on the Interface between Psychiatry and Anthropology. In: I. Galdston (Ed.): The Interface between Psychiatry and Anthropology. New York: Brunner/Mazel; London: Butterworths.

World Health Organization (1973): Report of The International Pilot Study of Schizophrenia. Volume 1. Geneva: WHO.

World Health Organization (1979): Report of the International Pilot Study of Schizophrenia. Volume 2. Chichester: John Wiley & Sons.

www.ingramcontent.com/pod-product-compliance
Ingram Content Group UK Ltd.
Pitfield, Milton Keynes, MK11 3LW, UK
UKHW020117290926
15471UKWH00003B/198

9 783820 469011